Remote Interpreting in Healthcare Settings

NEW TRENDS IN TRANSLATION STUDIES

Volume 34

Series Editor:
Professor Jorge Díaz Cintas

Advisory Board:
Professor Susan Bassnett
Professor Lynne Bowker
Professor Frederic Chaume
Professor Aline Remael

PETER LANG
Oxford • Bern • Berlin • Bruxelles • New York • Wien

Remote Interpreting in Healthcare Settings

Esther de Boe

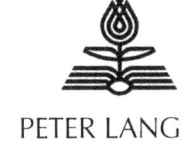

PETER LANG
Oxford • Bern • Berlin • Bruxelles • New York • Wien

Bibliographic information published by Die Deutsche Nationalbibliothek.
Die Deutsche Nationalbibliothek lists this publication in the Deutsche National-
bibliografie; detailed bibliographic data is available on the Internet at
http://dnb.d-nb.de.

A catalogue record for this book is available from the British Library.

Library of Congress Cataloging-in-Publication Data

Names: De Boe, Esther, 1971– author.
Title: Remote interpreting in healthcare settings / Esther de Boe.
Description: Oxford ; New York : Peter Lang, [2023] | Series: New trends in
  translation studies, 1664-249X ; volume no. 34 | Includes
  bibliographical references and index.
Identifiers: LCCN 2022024433 (print) | LCCN 2022024434 (ebook) | ISBN
  9781800793736 (paperback) | ISBN 9781800793743 (ebook) | ISBN
  9781800793750 (epub)
Subjects: LCSH: Health facilities—Translating services—Technological
  innovations. | Medicine—Translating. | Telecommunication in medicine. |
  Telephone interpreting.
Classification: LCC R119.5 .D43 2023 (print) | LCC R119.5 (ebook) | DDC
  362.1028—dc23/eng/20220720
LC record available at https://lccn.loc.gov/2022024433
LC ebook record available at https://lccn.loc.gov/2022024434

Cover design by Peter Lang Ltd.

ISSN 1664-249X
ISBN 978-1-80079-373-6 (print)
ISBN 978-1-80079-374-3 (ePDF)
ISBN 978-1-80079-375-0 (ePub)

© Peter Lang AG 2023

Published by Peter Lang Ltd, International Academic Publishers,
Oxford, United Kingdom
oxford@peterlang.com, www.peterlang.com

Esther de Boe has asserted her right under the Copyright, Designs and Patents Act, 1988, to be identified as Author of this Work.

All rights reserved.
All parts of this publication are protected by copyright.
Any utilisation outside the strict limits of the copyright law, without
the permission of the publisher, is forbidden and liable to prosecution.
This applies in particular to reproductions, translations, microfilming,
and storage and processing in electronic retrieval systems.

This publication has been peer reviewed.

Contents

List of Figures   ix

List of Tables   xi

Acknowledgements   xiii

List of Abbreviations   xv

Transcription Key   xvii

PART I   Remote Interpreting   1

CHAPTER 1
Introduction   3
- 1.1 Interpreting and technology   3
- 1.2 Methods of remote interpreting   4
- 1.3 The advance of remote interpreting   7
- 1.4 Research design   10
- 1.5 Structure of this book   13

CHAPTER 2
What Do We Know about RI?   15
- 2.1 Remote conference interpreting   15
- 2.2 Remote dialogue interpreting   23
- 2.3 Research issues and caveats   54

PART II Theoretical Framework   57

CHAPTER 3
Investigating Quality   59
3.1 Interpreting quality   59
3.2 Remote healthcare interpreting: A holistic approach   69

CHAPTER 4
Methodology   73
4.1 General outline and research questions   73
4.2 Data collection   76
4.3 Annotation   86
4.4 Analysis   95

PART III Results   107

CHAPTER 5
Miscommunication and Interaction Management   109
5.1 Message equivalence issues   110
5.2 Interactional issues   123
5.3 Interaction management   128
5.4 Concurrence   131

CHAPTER 6
Challenges to Communication Quality   133
6.1 Series 1   134
6.2 Series 2   156
6.3 Series 3   174

CHAPTER 7
Participant Perceptions — 187
- 7.1 Post-simulation interviews — 188
- 7.2 Retrospective interviews — 202

CHAPTER 8
Conclusion and Discussion — 211
- 8.1 Summary research objectives and questions — 211
- 8.2 Miscommunication — 214
- 8.3 Interaction management — 217
- 8.4 Main communication challenges in RI — 220
- 8.5 Implications for interpreter practice and training — 233
- 8.6 Limitations of this study — 236
- 8.7 Suggestions for future research — 238

Bibliography — 241

Index — 263

Figures

Figure 1.	Terminological representation of spoken-language remote dialogue interpreting methods.	6
Figure 2.	Quality of remote dialogue interpreting.	60
Figure 3.	Example of empty annotation spreadsheet.	85
Figure 4.	Seating arrangement in VI-1.	192
Figure 5.	Seating arrangement in VI-2.	197
Figure 6.	Seating arrangement in VI-3.	201

Tables

Table 1.	Distribution of the scenarios across the series and conditions	79
Table 2a.	Basic scenario 1A, F2FI-1	79
Table 2b.	List of complaints scenario 1A, F2FI-1	80
Table 3.	Duration body (in minutes:seconds)	80
Table 4.	Duration opening (in minutes:seconds)	81
Table 5.	Duration closing (in minutes:seconds)	81
Table 6.	Overview of average full-turn length in body (in seconds and milliseconds)	82
Table 7.	Annotation model	88
Table 8.	Frequency of message equivalence issues	111
Table 9.	Types of message equivalence issues	112
Table 10.	Order of interpreting method vs. number of message equivalence issues	113
Table 11.	Frequency of interactional issues	124
Table 12.	Types of interactional issues	125
Table 13.	Frequency of repair and optimization strategies	129
Table 14.	Overview of types of repair and optimization strategies	130
Table 15.	Concurrence of issues	132
Table 16.	Duration of openings and closings, Series 1 (in minutes:seconds)	151
Table 17.	Duration of openings and closings, Series 2 (in minutes:seconds)	171
Table 18.	Duration of openings and closings, Series 3 (in minutes:seconds)	184

Acknowledgements

Writing this book has been a highly instructive, challenging and enjoyable experience, for which I would like to thank everyone who has supported me in various ways over the past few years.

First of all, I would like to thank Peter Lang International Academic Publishers, in particular, Professor Jorge Díaz-Cintas, for providing me with the wonderful opportunity to publish this book, and Dr Laurel Plapp for her kind support during the editing process.

I would also like to thank the University of Antwerp's Department of Applied Linguistics, Translation & Interpreting, in particular the French section – Prof. Katrien Lievois, Prof. Isabelle Robert and Prof. Kris Peeters – for their support in starting a PhD.

I am also extremely grateful to my dear PhD advisors from the University of Antwerp – Prof. Emerita Aline Remael and Prof. Jim Ureel – for the many hours they spent on reading my work and for always providing me with constructive feedback and kind support. For her specialized advice, I would also very much like to thank my PhD advisor from the University of Surrey, Prof. Sabine Braun.

I greatly appreciated the help from all the participants in the simulations, who have been indispensable in collecting the data for this research: the three interpreters, who were brave enough to expose themselves to the critical analyses of their performances, and the simulated patients. I am also immensely grateful to Dr Irene van der Avoort, who was willing to volunteer as a gynaecologist in all nine simulations, and to Dr Jan van der Avoort, for his professional advice on the gynaecological themes.

Lastly, I would especially like to thank my beloved parents, my brother and sister and their partners, as well as my friends, who all provided such great support along the way and were always there for me. Special thanks go to my loving partner, Kris, for his infinite words of encouragement, his patience and all his love. And last but not least, I would like to thank my daughter Anaïs, my little ray of sunshine, whose smiles, hugs and laughter bring me so much happiness.

Abbreviations

CAI	computer-assisted interpreting
DI	dialogue interpreting
ET	environment and technology
F2FI	face-to-face interpreting
IA issue	interactional issue
IA management	interaction management
ME	message equivalence
MI	machine interpreting
RCI	remote conference interpreting
RDI	remote dialogue interpreting
RI	remote interpreting
RO	repair and optimization
TCI	teleconference interpreting
TI	telephone interpreting
TRI	telephone remote interpreting
VCI	videoconference interpreting
VI	video interpreting
VRI	video remote interpreting

Transcription Key

Transcription conventions

80	Turn number
(D)	Doctor
(P)	Patient
(I)	Interpreter
Bold	issues at the level of message equivalence and interaction discussed in the analysis are marked in **bold**
<u>**Bold + underscore**</u>	overlapping speech; the overlapping utterances are aligned vertically, e.g.: (D) What do you mean <u>**exactly**</u>? (I) <u>**What do you**</u> mean exactly?
[*xyz*]	Extralinguistic information, e.g. [*laugh*], [*French*]
[xyz]	Participant utterance, e.g., [that's right] or short audible expression, e.g., [hm m] during another participant's turn
()	Non-floor taking turn by a participant that occurs within another participant's turn
(.)	Pause length, values between short (.) and longer (..) (…)
[…]	A less relevant part of the excerpt has been omitted to avoid unnecessarily long examples
..	Unfinished phrase

PART I

Remote Interpreting

CHAPTER 1

Introduction

This chapter situates the topic under investigation – remote interpreting (RI) – in a broader context by providing background information on the use of technology in the field of interpreting (Section 1.1) and types of RI methods (Section 1.2). It also discusses reasons for the growing use of RI in today's society, as well as the outcomes of previous RI research, demonstrating the need for the current research (Section 1.3). Subsequently, the design of this research will be outlined (Section 1.4), as well as the structure of this book (Section 1.5).

1.1 Interpreting and technology

In only a relatively short span of time, technology has profoundly affected the way we communicate. Especially since the outbreak of the COVID-19 pandemic in 2020, the use of communication technology has boomed. However, even before the worldwide health crisis, technological developments had already started to have a significant impact on the fields of translation and interpreting and will continue to do so exponentially. For interpreting, Fantinuoli (2018: 2–3) distinguishes three major technological breakthroughs. The first one was the introduction of wired systems for speech transmission, allowing for simultaneous interpreting (SI). This technology enabled interpreters to render translations of speeches at the same time as speakers delivered them. Given that before that time, interpreting was carried out consecutively, that is, after speakers had (partly) finished their speeches, the introduction of SI produced massive time savings. The second breakthrough was the arrival of the internet, which all of a sudden provided interpreters with access to vast sources of information. This hugely facilitated the ways in which interpreters could prepare for assignments and make use of resources during assignments. As a third breakthrough, Fantinuoli (2018) mentions the introduction of interpreting-related technologies, that is, computer-assisted interpreting (CAI), machine interpreting (MI) and remote interpreting (RI). These technologies constitute a "technological turn" in interpreting, since they have the potential of radically transforming the interpreting profession (*ibid.*: 3). Whereas CAI is supposed to facilitate the interpreting task and MI potentially attempts to replace the human interpreter, RI technology changes the ways in which interpreting services are delivered. Before elaborating on the rise of RI and its impact, I will first clarify some of the key concepts related to its different constellations.

1.2 Methods of remote interpreting

Traditionally, interpreting services were delivered exclusively by means of face-to-face interpreting (F2FI; also called "in-person", "onsite" or "traditional" interpreting). However, as discussed in the previous section, contemporary communication channels allow for various methods of RI (also called "distance interpreting"), carried out by means of telephone (telephone interpreting; TI) or video link (video interpreting; VI).

To limit the scope of the rapidly expanding and heterogeneous field of research on RI, the overview of RI constellations provided here is restricted to spoken language, interpersonal interpreter-mediated communication (as opposed to mass communication, such as press conferences). Interpersonal interpreting is characterized by a direct relationship between the participants (Braun, 2006: 3) and can be divided into "monologic" and "dialogue" interpreting (Pöchhacker, 2004: 16). In monologic constellations, the primary participants are the speakers and their audiences (e.g. conference situations, formal meetings or debates with multilingual teams of interpreters), and interpreters usually work (in a booth) from their

Introduction 5

B- or C-language into their A-language, most frequently in the simultaneous mode (Braun, 2006: 3). By contrast, dialogue interpreting (DI), the context under investigation in this research, is considered a "three-party interaction" (Anderson, 1976/2002), with an interpreter assuming the pivotal, mediating role between two clients (Pöchhacker, 2004: 16). In such environments, the interpreter generally works in both language directions and in consecutive or (whispered) simultaneous mode (Braun, 2006: 3).

As is common in fields that lack systematic research, the terminology used to denote RI is far from consistent. Early definitions are marked by the predominance of conference interpreting in this field at the time. Mouzourakis (1996) and Niska (1999) proposed a series of definitions based on those used by AIIC (Association Internationale des Interprètes de Conférence, the international association of conference interpreters), defining RI as "simultaneous interpreting where the interpreter is not in the same room as the speaker or his/her audience" (Mouzourakis, 1996: 22–23; Niska, 1999: 110–111). In more recent denominations, the communication's mediated character is emphasized by the use of the term "video-mediated interpreting" or VMI (Braun, 2012).

For the purpose of the research presented in this work, the more general RI definition given by Ko (2006: 325) will be used as an umbrella term to cover all types of distance interpreting:

> The mode of interpreting in which the interpreter and the people being interpreted for (i.e., the clients) do not meet face-to-face and interpreting is conducted via media such as the telephone, the Internet, videoconferencing and other forms of telecommunications technology that enable interpreting to take place.

In this work, a further distinction is made between settings of conference interpreting and settings of dialogue interpreting. When RI takes place in a conference setting, the term "remote conference interpreting" (RCI) (Braun, 2007: 21) applies, whereas we will refer to RI in dialogue interpreting settings as "remote dialogue interpreting" (RDI). The latter type of RI is central to the current research. The various constellations of spoken-language remote dialogue interpreting are represented in Figure 1.

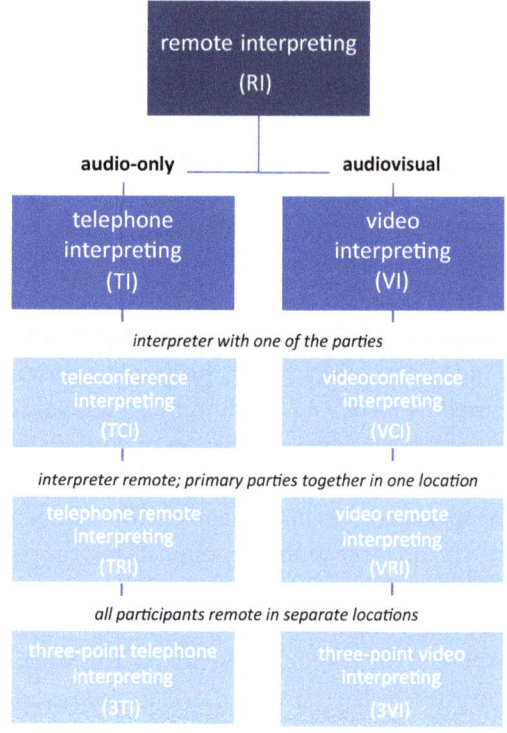

Figure 1. Terminological representation of spoken-language remote dialogue interpreting methods.

Figure 1 is based on the general distinction by Kelly (2008) between, on the one hand, "telephone interpretation" or "over-the-phone interpreting" (Braun, 2015) and, on the other, "video interpretation", also known as "video-link interpreting" (Hlavac, 2013) or "video-mediated interpreting" (Braun, 2018). Throughout this work, these two main types of RI will be referred to as telephone interpreting (TI) and video interpreting (VI).

The two main types of RI are divided into further subcategories. Within VI, a distinction is made between "videoconference interpreting" (VCI) and "video remote interpreting" (VRI), as described by Braun and Taylor (2012a). In VCI, the proceedings take place in two different, video-linked locations, while the interpreter is present with one of the parties, whereas in VRI, the interpreter works from a remote location (*ibid.*: 39–41). It must be noted that the term "VRI" also refers to a type of RI used to convey sign language (Mouzourakis, 2006: 46).

Telephone interpreting (TI) refers to situations in which the interpreter works over the telephone, either at the same location as one of the interlocutors or at a separate location (Lee, 2007: 231). In analogy to VI, TI can be subdivided based on a similar distinction, with teleconference interpreting (TCI) being the interpreting method in which the interpreter is present at the same location as one of the primary parties, and telephone remote interpreting (TRI) the one in which the interpreter works from a remote location.

A third constellation that is increasingly being used, especially since the principle of social distancing came along due to the COVID-19 pandemic, is one in which all participants (including the interpreter) are communicating from remote locations and connected via telephone or video link. This is referred to as "three-point TI" and "three-point VI", respectively.

The methods used in the simulations that provided the data for this book were TRI and VRI. In other words, for both RI methods, the primary participants (the doctor and the patient) were together in one location, whereas the interpreter was connected from a remote location. For the sake of simplicity, the terms "TI" and "VI" will be used to refer to the interpreting methods used for the simulations in this work. In the literature review (Chapter 2), constellations will be specified when relevant.

1.3 The advance of remote interpreting

So far, I have discussed the technological advances that allowed for the introduction of RI. This section is concerned with the societal context that enabled its expansion. As our societies become increasingly multilingual and multicultural, the demand in interpreting services continues to grow (Tipton & Furmanek, 2016). Moreover, the demand for language combinations has been come extremely varied. As a result of this growing and varied demand, interpreting services can no longer be realistically offered by F2FI only (González Rodríguez & Spinolo, 2017: 242). This is where RI comes in as an alternative to counter imbalances between demand and supply and ensure language mediation, as an example, for minorities. In this way, the use of RI enhances the access to public services by non-native speakers. Moreover, awareness for technology-mediated interpreting has increased as a result of new legislation in the legal context, since the European Directive 2010/64/EU on the right to interpretation and translation in criminal proceedings explicitly mentions the use of communication technologies to improve access to qualified legal interpreters (Skinner et al., 2018: 13). Moreover, in many Western countries, governments are legally obligated to cover the cost of interpreting services, for example, in public service settings (*ibid.*: 14). This also pushes the demand for interpreting services and the need to increase access, which can be facilitated by RI. Also, as Spinolo et al. (2018a: 46) point out, RI fits in with some of the main objectives of the European Digital Agenda, such as improving digital skills and generating social benefits by using communication technology to reduce energy consumption and optimize healthcare and other public services.

As a result, RI contributes to a higher productivity in interpreting in the form of an increased demand for interpreting services (Fantinuoli, 2018: 7). RI offers numerous benefits to clients and interpreters, such as a greater access to the global labour market and to users, the protection of clients' and interpreters' privacy, as well as more flexible working hours for interpreters, with the possibility of working from home (Spinolo et al., 2018b: 12). However, as Braun (2018: 416) puts forward, RI is "more than a technical solution, but a complex social practice". As such, the use of RI is often problematized, for example, as far as interpreting quality is concerned. Ever since the first RI experiments were conducted, ensuring quality in RI has been the subject of heated debate (Spinolo et al., 2018b: 22), especially among interpreters. Also, the impact of the use of RI methods on interpreters' working conditions remains a major issue, which not only concerns the ergonomic aspects of screen work, but also the emotional and social aspects of the interpreter's virtual instead of physical participation to the communication (Alley, 2012; Napier et al., 2018). Besides, the use of RI is also often criticized as a means of cutting costs at the expense of the interpreter (Tipton & Furmanek, 2016: 143).

As it is, interpreting, in its many forms and constellations, is considered an extremely challenging cognitive task (Gile, 1995). On top of that, the different contexts that interpreters face in their professional practice often require highly specialized knowledge of a specific setting and corresponding terminology. For example, in healthcare settings, the accuracy of the interpretation is the most critical component of safe and effective communication between healthcare providers and patients (Anazawa et al., 2012). When the interpreting takes place while one or more interlocutors and/or the interpreter are not physically present, but participate remotely, this adds another layer of complexity to the interpreting process (Braun, 2006, 2013; Braun & Davitti, 2018; Braun & Taylor, 2012a; Napier & Leneham, 2011). This has come to the fore in previous research on RI, as discussed in Chapter 2.

Despite its potentially problematic character, the different constellations of RI are rapidly gaining a firm footing in the practice of interpreting and have therefore also become an increasingly researched subject within interpreting studies. Whereas early studies on RI focused on remote conference interpreting (RCI), various areas of DI such as court interpreting, healthcare interpreting and business interpreting are being investigated more and more. Pioneer research on TI was carried out by Wadensjö (1999), who compared police interviews conducted face-to-face and by telephone. In the field of VI, Braun (2003, 2004) and Braun and Kohn (2001) conducted ground-breaking fieldwork in business interpreting settings.

Notwithstanding the growing body of research on RI, the subject is still under-represented in the field of interpreting studies, as are other domains of technology-mediated interpreting (Fantinuoli, 2018). Most of the RI research in interpreting studies has been conducted in the legal context (Braun & Taylor, 2012a). Other fields of DI, such as healthcare interpreting, have so far remained under-exposed in interpreting studies, and have predominantly been investigated in medical studies focussing on patient satisfaction and quality of care (Pöchhacker, 2006). Moreover, only a few studies have engaged in micro-analytic studies of the nature of RI methods (Napier et al., 2018).

Empirical research on RI usually compares different methods of interpreting: face-to-face interpreting and RI methods performed by means of different channels (audio-only or audiovisual), which are tested in a specific setting (e.g. conference, medical, business or legal). Within this empirical research, we can distinguish between research based on subjective testing measures (e.g. interviews, surveys), aimed at examining users' perceptions and satisfaction, and research based on objective assessments, with the purpose of identifying typical features of RI and establishing the influence of the remote conditions on the communicative situation (Castagnoli & Niemants, 2018).

As is typical of research topics that incorporate several disciplines, the empirical studies on RI are widely divergent in many respects, such as research design, scale, definitions and methods used. As a result, we still know relatively little about which characteristics of RI can be considered common across all contexts and which features tend to depend on other factors, such as the specific setting, interpreting constellation, the interpreter's experience and the language combination. Moreover, in interpreting studies, research has focused mostly on either TI or VI, but so far, no studies have compared different RI methods with F2FI. With my research, I attempt to fill this gap by comparing RI across three different interpreting methods in simulated healthcare settings, as I will explain in Section 1.4.

1.4 Research design

This research makes a qualitative comparison of interpreter-mediated healthcare communication across three different interpreting methods: (1) face-to-face interpreting (F2FI), (2) telephone interpreting (TI) and (3) video interpreting (VI). By comparing these three methods, I investigate possible differences in the quality of the communication and make an attempt to establish to what extent such differences may be attributed to the remote conditions.

To allow for a systematic comparison between the different interpreting methods, I designed a methodology that was based on three series of simulated interpreter-mediated doctor–patient consultations. Compared with authentic data, simulations have the clear advantage that they allow for

Introduction

a highly controlled environment with comparable conditions. Within each series of simulations, a professional female interpreter performed her task using three interpreting methods (F2FI, TI and VI) in the consecutive mode. After each simulation, the participants were questioned about their perceptions of (1) the quality of the interpreting, (2) the quality of the communication, (3) the quality of the healthcare provided, (4) their satisfaction with the technical conditions and the seating arrangement and (5) their preferences with regard to the different interpreting methods. All simulations were video recorded by means of several cameras each with a different angle to cover all of the interaction.

For the purpose of the data analysis, the concept of quality was operationalized based on a literature review. This review identified two key components to quality, that is, message equivalence and interaction management. These two components constitute the basis of measuring quality, since they represent, on the one hand, the quality of the interpreting in terms of accuracy or correspondence between the source text and the target text (message equivalence), and, on the other, indicate how the interaction was collaboratively coordinated by the participants (interaction management). Based on this insight, a taxonomy for measuring quality was designed and applied to the corpus. After this, an extensive investigation of the relationships between the different categories was carried out by looking into communication issues in terms of message equivalence, interaction management and technological factors.

Across the two RI methods, I examined possible benefits and drawbacks of adding image to the audio channel by looking into potential differences. This is of particular importance to healthcare interpreting, where the number of interpreting services carried out by VI is growing, for example, in the form of intercultural mediation by video link (Verrept, 2011; Verrept & Coune, 2016). As such, they increasingly replace traditional F2FI and TI services, especially in large hospital campuses (Tipton & Furmanek, 2016). Finally, the results from the comparative, qualitative analysis of the simulations were triangulated with the findings of the subjective assessment by means of a qualitative analysis of the participants' perceptions.

The conceptual approach to interpreting adopted in this study is in line with the so-called "dialogic discourse-based interactionist paradigm"

(Pöchhacker, 2016: 75) in interpreting studies. This paradigm views the interpreting process as a constructive and collaborative activity by all participants, including the interpreter, who are in a continuous process of negotiating meaning (Baraldi & Gavioli, 2012; Bot, 2005; Roy, 2000; Wadensjö, 1998). The study also acknowledges the multimodal character of human communication, which means that participants interacting with each other do so by using a multitude of verbal and nonverbal communicative resources to convey meaning and monitor comprehension (Mondada, 2016; Pasquandrea, 2011). At the same time, insights generated by research on RI within medical science and bilingual healthcare communication are also included in the conceptual framework.

Following this holistic approach, the results from the data analyses are meant to provide a clear picture of the shifts in quality that we may expect in technology-mediated healthcare interpreting, as well as clues about the role of technology in the interactional dynamics between the participants. The study therefore wants to shed critical light on three distinct features of interpreter-mediated communication related to the quality of the communication: (1) number and types of miscommunication, (2) causes of miscommunication, including technological and environmental factors, and (3) ways in which participants cope with miscommunication across the three different interpreting methods (F2FI, TI and VI).

The knowledge generated by the outcomes of this study will be extremely useful to all practitioners of RI, especially in the medical field, where there is still a dearth of evidence-based knowledge on the impact of the use of various RI methods on the quality of the communication between healthcare providers and patients. A more profound knowledge of potential challenges of RI to the quality of communication may help healthcare interpreters, providers and patients to anticipate to possible communication issues and be more proactive in adopting strategies to cope with these.

A better understanding of RI will also support interpreter trainers in preparing their students for the professional market, in which RI skills are indispensable. Furthermore, the results of this research are essential to other stakeholders concerned with RI, such as dedicated platforms providing RI services, who can learn from the analysis of participants' experiences with RI and adapt their supportive software accordingly. Next to that, this research is highly relevant to healthcare policy makers in order to take informed decisions on a responsible use of RI in their organizations and develop RI guidelines.

Finally, by exploring interpreter-mediated communication at a linguistic, interactional and multimodal level, it is hoped that this research contributes to our understanding of remote interpreted doctor–patient communication. The results of this investigation will produce a deeper awareness of possible changes in interactional processes in RI compared with F2FI and, in this way, contribute to the burgeoning body of research in various disciplines concerned with technology-mediated human interaction.

As opposed to previous research on remote dialogue interpreting, which was carried out from an exclusively medical or interpreting studies perspective, the present study adopts a more holistic, multidisciplinary approach by combining insights from medical science, interpreting studies and bilingual healthcare communication. This makes the study a unique project that could not be timelier in an era where many of us struggle to come to terms with the challenges of technology-mediated communication.

1.5 Structure of this book

This book consists of three parts. The first part is dedicated to what RI is, as explained in this first chapter and takes stock of what we already know about RI (Chapter 2), by looking into research carried out on this topic in a wider range of settings, discussing research results and methods relevant to my investigation into the impact of RI on the quality of communication in healthcare settings. Chapter 2 also identifies the gap in our knowledge on remote healthcare interpreting, demonstrating the need for my research. Subsequently, Part II (consisting of Chapters 3 and 4) provides the methodological framework of my research. In Chapter 3, I elaborate on the concepts that are essential to this research, such as interpreting quality, message equivalence and interaction management. This conceptual framework underpins the methodology, explained in Chapter 4, which presents the research design, research questions and objectives, as well as a description of how the data were collected and analysed. This is followed by the presentation of the results from the analyses in Part III, that starts with a discussion of miscommunication and interaction management observed in the simulations in Chapter 5 and zooms in into specific challenges of RI to communication quality in Chapter 6, by means of qualitative analyses of salient excerpts taken from the simulations. These analyses are triangulated by the participants' perceptions of communication quality in Chapter 7. Finally, Chapter 8 presents the overall conclusions of the research, a summary of the greatest challenges of RI and their implications for interpreting practice and training, as well as directions for future research.

CHAPTER 2

What Do We Know about RI?

This chapter takes stock of what we already know about remote interpreting by discussing the empirical research that has been carried out on this topic. Although the scope of this work is remote dialogue interpreting (RDI), the literature review starts with a discussion of some of the findings from research on remote conference interpreting (RCI, Section 2.1), since this research dates back to long before the first studies on RDI were initiated and many of its results are relevant to the current research. I will then zoom in to the central research theme of this work by providing an overview of studies on RDI (Section 2.2). Empirical research on RDI has been carried out from the perspective of medical science, on the one hand, and of interpreting studies, on the other, each with very different research angles. Since this makes a direct comparison of the findings from these studies difficult, research from the two disciplines is discussed in separate sections, starting with medial studies in Section 2.2.1, followed by interpreting studies in Section 2.2.2. This literature review is by no means exhaustive, but focuses on aspects that are relevant to the present research.

2.1 Remote conference interpreting

The first studies on RI were implemented in the context of conference interpreting, that is, in interpreting situations in which all primary participants (of a multilingual conference, meeting or debate) are in the same room, and the interpreters work from a separate location (Braun,

2007: 22), either by a cabled arrangement[1] or via a videoconferencing set-up (Moser-Mercer, 2003: 1). The earliest experiments – based on satellite transmission of image and sound, which made them extremely costly – took place in the 1970s. Examples of these are UNESCO's Paris–Nairobi "Symphonie Satellite" conference (Andres & Falk, 2009; Moser-Mercer, 2005b; Mouzourakis, 1996; Thiéry, 1976), the United Nations' 1978 New York–Buenos Aires test (Chernov, 2004; Moser-Mercer, 2005b) and a similar test during a United Nations conference in Vienna in 1982 (Andres & Falk, 2009). When asked about the perception of their performance, interpreters complained of an increase in stress and fatigue and the lack of social presence. These issues were mainly attributed to the interpreters' limited view of the speaker and the audience (Ziegler & Gigliobianco, 2018: 120). Moreover, the interpreters were not satisfied with their performance and the technology was considered too expensive by the users (Andres & Falk, 2009: 11; Kurz, 2000: 100).

Technological innovations such as ISDN (Integrated Services Digital Network) and cable connections (Mouzourakis, 2006) made RCI cheaper and more accessible. Early research with this "new" technology was highly experimental, including the exploratory study by ETSI (European Telecommunications Standards Institute) in co-operation with the AIIC Technical Committee in 1992. Its objective was to identify

> the special videoconference requirements of conference interpreters and to establish whether ISDN [...] video telephony offers a sufficient audio bandwidth and image quality to support interpreters in their work. (Niska, 1999: 115)

The conclusion of the ETSI/AIIC study was that lower levels of video and audio bandwidth did not support simultaneous interpretation. Given the existing technological standards at the time, RCI by means of ISDN video telephony caused increased fatigue and lower interpreter

---

1   In the past, RI took place via satellite. However, it is now usually performed by using terrestrial telephone lines, either ISDN (Integrated Services Digital Network) lines, or direct cable (coaxial and fibre optics) connections between the conference room and the remote cabins within the same building complex. For detailed technical specifications, see Mouzourakis (1996, 2006).

satisfaction with their performance. This was confirmed in a similar test by AIIC in 1997 (Kurz, 2000; Niska, 1999). However, as Gile (1992, in Niska, 1999: 119) points out, it must be kept in mind that although the acoustic quality of these early set-ups was poor, affecting interpreting quality and causing fatigue and stress, "in non-remote interpreting, be it cabled or wireless, acoustic problems [are] not a rare occurrence either".

The use of so-called new technologies experienced a boom at the beginning of the 1990s (Andres & Falk, 2009). With the expansion of the European Union, the institutions in Brussels started to look for cost-effective ways of dealing with the space constraints caused by the increasing number of interpreters and conducted a number of tests with RCI for that specific purpose. Interpreters were set up in centralized interpreter hubs with video screens providing them with audio and video from the actual meeting rooms (Braun & Taylor, 2012a: 34–35). Other experiments were conducted by the European Commission in 1995, 1997, 2000 and 2010 (Braun & Taylor, 2012a), as well as by the European Parliament in 2001 and the European Council in 1999 and 2001, in collaboration with the United Nations (Moser-Mercer, 2005b). In an overview, Mouzourakis (2006) lists eleven RCI experiments in conference settings, conducted between 1990 and 2004, mainly discussing technical features, such as the technical requirements for sound and image transmission, image capture and display and meeting room views. It concludes that during the testing, the major disadvantage of RCI was the unavoidable loss of visual information (*ibid.*: 6).

The importance of visual information is also reflected in the ISO standards[2] developed for RCI, which define minimum working conditions for conference interpreters working remotely in permanent or mobile booths. These standards are adopted by, among others, the International Association of Conference interpreters (AIIC), the European Court of Justice and the European Parliament (Ziegler & Gigliobianco, 2018). According to the standards, interpreters must have a direct view of the speaker and the

---

2   Details of current ISO standards (2020) can be found in the AIIC Reference Guide for Remote Simultaneous Interpreting: <https://aiic.ch/wp-content/uploads/2020/05/aiic-ch-reference-guide-to-rsi.pdf>.

conference room (AIIC, 2000: 2) and receive high-definition images of the speakers and the participants (Ziegler & Gigliobianco, 2018: 128).

The importance of visual communication signals for conference interpreters was investigated earlier by Bühler (1985) by means of a survey and a series of interviews. She found that interpreters objected to RI because of "a general feeling of discomfort or undue stress", although they found it difficult to specify the precise reasons for their objections. This could be explained by the fact that nonverbal signals are mostly perceived unconsciously and "often become apparent only by their absence" (Bühler, 1985: 50). Bühler (*ibid.*) concluded that visual information is important for conference interpreters with regard to non-vocal signals from the speakers and the conference delegates, in the context of social interaction between the conference participants and the interpreter and among conference interpreters. This led her to conclude that "any impairment of the natural multichannel communication situation is highly undesirable" in conference interpreting (*ibid.*: 53). In another small-scale controlled experiment by Kurz (1996) among student interpreters, the lack of visual input was also perceived to have a negative impact on feelings of social presence, fatigue and performance. Nevertheless, other studies on the role of visual information in conference interpreting using a matched design (Anderson, 1994; Balzani, 1990; Tommola & Lindholm, 1995) showed little or no significant decline in performance during tests comparing "video-on" and "video-off" interpreting methods. Moreover, Bacigalupe (1999) put the importance of vision into perspective by describing the physical conditions in live conference interpreting, emphasizing that conference rooms are often so big that it is impossible to clearly see the speaker from the interpreting posts. Bacigalupe (*ibid.*) also highlights that interpreters frequently cover their faces with their hands when they try to concentrate on the content of the message, and often focus on audiovisual material in the room rather than on the speaker. In his empirical study on the relevance of visual contact between interpreter and speaker, the hypothesis that visual contact improves the interpreter's performance was not confirmed. However, Bacigalupe (*ibid.*: 135) emphasizes that

> in spite of these results, visual input seems to be essential for contextualization of the "physical" situation where the speech is delivered: Who is speaking? Who is going

to speak next? Is it a man or a woman? are questions easily answered by means of visual information and a necessary source of input for a successful interpretation.

Similarly, Moser-Mercer (2005a: 730) argues that visual information plays a crucial role in the complex "multisensory integration" humans use to infer the intended meaning of a spoken message from its context. In comparison with the reality of a conference room, the visual information in RCI is often inadequate, forcing interpreters to develop new communication strategies (*ibid.*: 737).

The first controlled experiment that assessed both technical and human factors in RCI (psychological and medical aspects, information processing from multiple sources, operation of multiple controls, motivation and social isolation) was a test in Geneva in 1999 by ETI (École de Traduction et d'Interprétation), ITU (International Telecommunications Union) and Swisscom. This study investigated interpreters' psychological and physiological responses to remote versus "normal" interpreting (Moser-Mercer, 2005a: 75; Mouzourakis, 2006: 63). It concluded that, for interpreters, working face-to-face in a conference room is psychologically less stressful, less tiring and leads to better interpreting performance (ITU/ETI/Swisscom, 1999: 19). Nevertheless, saliva samples indicating the level of stress hormones, taken before and after the tests, did not show a substantial difference between the levels of stress hormones of interpreters in the booth inside the conference room and those doing RCI (Andres & Falk, 2009: 12). Yet, the interpreters complained of physiological troubles such as sore eyes, back and neck pain, headaches and nausea. They also had psychological complaints, for example, loss of concentration and motivation (Mouzourakis, 2006: 52). These issues may have been related to the remote interpreters' feelings of "alienation" or "absence of a feeling of presence in the meeting room, universally experienced by interpreters under RI conditions" (*ibid.*: 45). Even in extremely good technical conditions, remote conference interpreters experienced more fatigue and stress and had a number of physiological and psychological complaints (*ibid.*: 52–53).

The notion of "social presence", that is, the feeling of being in the same room with the speaker and the ability to form an impression of the speaker (Kurz, 1996: 7) or the absence thereof, is also referred to as "absence of a feeling of participation", "interpreter alienation" (Mouzourakis, 2006: 56) and "isolation from the real world" (Moser-Mercer, 2005a: 732). This notion is much evoked in the literature on RCI. Moser-Mercer (2005b: 78) claims that the feeling of a lack of presence, combined with cognitive overload, leads to fatigue and thus to poorer performance in RCI compared with F2FI and goes hand in hand with the feeling of a lack of control. Aside from fatigue, feelings of lack of presence and control, and cognitive overload, other problems experienced by remote conference interpreters in the aforementioned tests were lack of feedback from the audience, greater tension and nervousness (Kurz, 1999: 115).

The largest and most comprehensive experimental study on RCI was carried out in 2004 by the European Parliament. Its main objective was to examine the possible repercussions for interpreters working in RCI compared to interpreters performing "onsite" conference interpreting (Mertens-Hoffman, 2005, in Roziner & Shlesinger, 2010). The study is the first one in this field to draw attention to the role of attitude and psychological factors in interpreters' acceptance of RI. Although the remote conditions had a relatively small impact on interpreting quality and interpreters' health and objective measures of stress, the results also showed that the remote conditions had considerable psychological effects on interpreters, such as an increase in feelings of isolation and alienation (Roziner & Shlesinger, 2010: 214). The study revealed a discrepancy between the negative self-assessment of interpreters during RCI and the much less negative objective outcomes of their performance (*ibid.*: 216).

As Mouzourakis (2006: 45) highlighted, most of the RCI experiments were constrained by their specific settings, which undermines their validity to a certain degree and calls for "a more cohesive research methodology". Braun (2007: 23) also draws attention to the fact that the findings of the RCI experiments were closely linked to the experimental conditions, rendering the interpreting difficult and unfamiliar, which may have influenced the outcomes. Roziner and Shlesinger (2010: 218) share Braun's (2007) opinion when they consider that it may not be the fact of being removed from the work floor per se that is important, but rather the interpreters' expectation of a qualitative decline, which functions as a "self-fulfilling prophecy". This finding is confirmed by Gile (1992, in Niska, 1999: 120), who claims that interpreters' attitudes can represent a "non-negligible obstacle" in research measuring the pros and cons of RI and who considers the possibility that interpreters fearing RI will unconsciously perform less well in this interpreting method, whereas interpreters who are happy to use new technology may perform better.

Another discrepancy that was observed in the experiments was the gap between interpreters' and clients' perceptions of performance quality in RCI. Questionnaire data from RCI experiments revealed that clients, contrary to interpreters, were often satisfied with this interpreting method (Andres & Falk, 2009). Mouzourakis (1996: 32) explains the difference in perceptions of RCI by interpreters and non-interpreters using the argument that interpreters compared videoconferencing conditions to those of live simultaneous interpretation in regular meeting rooms and found the former inferior, whereas non-interpreters tend to compare videoconferencing conditions to the communication medium that was most known to them at the time, namely the telephone. As a result, for the interpreters, RCI was an inferior interpreting method compared with onsite conference interpreting, whereas for clients, it was superior compared to telephone conferencing.

A more recent experiment with RCI investigated the feasibility of different technological set-ups, including a 65-inch screen with a picture-in-picture function, a camera remotely controlled by the interpreter and a 360-degree camera combined with virtual reality (VR) glasses (Ziegler & Gigliobianco, 2018). The interpreters participating in the experiment were asked to share their opinions about the different solutions, especially about the quality of the technology used. Whereas the interpreters welcomed the picture-in-picture screen and the remotely controlled camera to compensate for the lack of a full view of the participants, their opinions about the operability of VR glasses combined with traditional equipment were mixed.

In light of the results of the empirical research on RCI, we can conclude that, despite the relatively positive experience of clients and the lack of objective proof of deterioration in quality, the remote interpreters participating in the research discussed above suffered from physiological and psychological complaints, compared with conference interpreters performing their tasks onsite. This was caused by a lack of visual information and social presence, enhancing the cognitive complexity of their assignments and leading to fatigue and feelings of alienation, loss of motivation and a lack of control. Therefore, most of the research insists on optimizing the external and technical conditions in which RCI takes place, to limit the negative effects of RCI (Shlesinger, 2009: 10). Moreover, the interpreters' negative attitudes towards RCI apparently played an important role in the perceived quality decline (Gile, 1992, in Niska, 1999: 120).

As far as technical circumstances are concerned, it must be remarked these are continuously improving. The European Union's Directorate-General for Interpretation (DG-SCIC), the largest conference interpreters' agency in the world, which provides interpreters for the EU institutions, has monitored videoconferencing equipment since 1998. Meanwhile, it has designed appropriate technical set-ups for RCI, which are fully compliant with the applicable RCI standards (Esteban Causo, 2012). As Ziegler and Gigliobianco (2018) put forward, the general conditions for RCI are changing constantly due to globalization, changing market needs, digitalization and the rapid development of information and communication technologies. The technological developments in particular may help to overcome the current shortcomings of RCI as experienced by interpreters, given that

> the availability of hardware and software for dynamic monitoring and controlling of important parameters, such as lip synchronization, latency, video resolution and frequency response, as well as network infrastructures that allow for simultaneous transmission of high definition video and high quality audio signals via the Internet, combined with latest video, virtual reality and augmented reality (AR) technologies might offer possibilities to overcome existing technological, physiological and psychological problems. (*ibid.*: 120)

However, as Moser-Mercer (2005b: 75) argues, while the costs and efforts associated with high-quality RI set-ups are likely to decrease as equipment becomes less expensive and technical support staff more experienced, human factors will become one of the most important issues to be explored in remote interpreting.

It is obvious that the worldwide pandemic has greatly accelerated the advance of RCI (Fantinuoli, 2022). However, since this development is extremely recent, no studies have been able yet to systematically investigate the exact impact on interpreting performance (Seeber & Fox, 2022).

For the latest developments in this domain, see Chapters 35 and 36 of the Handbook of Conference Interpreting (Mikasa & Tiselius, 2022).

Compared with RCI studies, in research on remote dialogue interpreting (RDI), which is discussed in Section 2.3, human factors are investigated much more prominently than technological factors.

2.2 Remote dialogue interpreting

Whereas RCI has established technological standards and technical set-ups are continuously being improved to the point where research is shifting to focus on human factors, in remote dialogue interpreting (RDI), there are currently no such standards. This may be due to the variety of settings and the much lesser degree of professionalization of dialogue interpreters, compared with conference interpreters. As we have seen, major recurring themes in RCI research are the optimization of the technological conditions and the possible effects of these conditions on the interpreter's cognitive processing and psychological and physical state, as well as the concomitant impact on the quality of the interpreting performance. In the empirical research on RDI, the interpreter's performance is an important theme as well. However, considering the triadic character of the interaction, interpreting performance is mostly examined within the context of the interactional dynamics of the interpreter-mediated dialogue.

As far as RDI is concerned, the investigated themes and research methods are closely tied to the research discipline. As explained in the beginning of this chapter, on the one hand, there is research from medical science (Section 2.2.1), centred on patient satisfaction and quality of care (Pöchhacker, 2006). On the other hand, there are studies from interpreting studies, that take a more communicative-oriented perspective and are often multidisciplinary studies, that is, drawing on methodology from interpreting studies, humanities, sociolinguistics, communication studies and pragmatics (Section 2.2.2).

2.2.1 Medical studies

In the field of medical science, empirical studies in RI compared different modes and/or methods of medical interpreting (and combinations thereof), such as face-to-face consecutive and remote consecutive interpreting, and simultaneous interpreting by telephone and by video link. Between 1996 and 2012, at least nineteen studies that examined the use of RI in medical settings were published in academic medical journals, including three overviews (Azarmina & Wallace, 2005; Corey et al., 2017; Masland et al., 2010). Most of the medical studies originate from the United States and reflect a more general trend that can be observed in research on cross-cultural communication in healthcare: It focuses on the impact of interpreting on healthcare services in terms of the quality of care, patient satisfaction and costs (Pöchhacker, 2006: 149).

All of these studies start by stating that due to the rising number of US residents with Limited English Proficiency (LEP), patients and healthcare providers are increasingly facing language barriers, which are considered to have a negative impact on access to healthcare services (Baker et al., 1996; Flores et al., 1998). Some studies argue that language barriers lessen patients' satisfaction with healthcare services (Baker et al., 1998; Carasquillo et al., 1999), whereas others emphasize that language barriers lead to higher healthcare costs, due to increased diagnostic testing and hospitalization (Hampers et al., 1999; Hampers & MacNulty, 2002). Some studies also describe the risks of using untrained interpreters in healthcare (Flores et al., 2003), as well as the lack of compliance of healthcare provision with legal requirements, when the implementation of federal and state laws requiring language services is hindered by "the scarcity of bilingual health care providers and prohibitive interpretation costs" (Masland et al., 2010: 739).

The main objective of these empirical medical studies is to seek ways to decrease language barriers and mitigate their negative impact through the use of new technology in the form of RI. As Locatis et al. (2011: 1) indicate,

> professional medical interpretation services have usually been provided in-person or by phone. Protocols have been developed enabling transmission of voice and video data over computer networks and increasing internet bandwidth has improved the prospects of offering [medical interpretation] services by video.

Another way to mitigate language barriers is to use professional interpreters instead of informal interpreters such as family members or untrained hospital personnel. Therefore, a large part of the medical research extends its scope beyond investigating the specific remote aspects of the communication and also compares professional versus informal (or ad hoc) interpreters and bilingual personnel, as well as so-called language-concordant and language-discordant groups. As a result, the outcomes of these studies are often also indicative of differences between professional (i.e. formal) and non-professional (i.e. informal) interpreting, as well as between interpreter-mediated and non-interpreted medical healthcare services.

Although the medical studies on RI address heterogeneous questions, a number of themes prevail, namely differences between RI and face-to-face interpreting (F2FI) in terms of consultation length and satisfaction (of patients, health care providers and interpreters), service quality (assessed by measuring audiovisual quality, accuracy, the number of utterances by each party, and subjective assessment), and costs for equipment and the professionals' time (Azarmina & Wallace, 2005). Of all these issues, the one most frequently researched by far is the effect of the interpreting method on patient satisfaction with the medical visit and the communication, often in combination with healthcare provider satisfaction and occasionally interpreter perceptions, mostly measured by means of post-test questionnaires.

The general outcomes of the medical studies on RI indicate patient satisfaction with different methods of RI (Crossman et al., 2010; Gany et al., 2007a, 2007b; Hornberger et al., 1996; Jones et al., 2003; Kuo & Fagan, 1999; Lee et al., 2002; Locatis et al., 2010, 2011; Nápoles et al., 2010; Paras et al., 2002; Price Leemann et al., 2012; Saint-Louis et al., 2003). Apart from Saint-Louis et al. (2003), in all studies, healthcare providers were as satisfied with RI as they were with F2FI. Saint-Louis et al. (2003: 51), who observed lower patient satisfaction among older and less educated persons, found that healthcare provider satisfaction was influenced by the age of the provider, the number of years of practice and their previous experience with F2FI.

Azarmina and Wallace (2005: 144), who reviewed nine studies on RI in medical communication carried out between 1996 and 2003, conclude that

> [...] the findings of the studies suggest that remote interpreting is at least as acceptable as physically present interpretation to patients, doctors and (to a lesser extent) interpreters themselves. Remote interpreting seems to be associated with levels of accuracy at least as good as those found in physically present interpretation, while offering potential cost savings. The latter, however, appear to depend on the volume of use of such services and the healthcare context.

Other positive features highlighted by Azarmina and Wallace's (2005: 144) review are the "ready access to qualified interpreters with a potentially wide range of language skills" and the finding that RI "significantly increases the efficiency of interpreters by reducing the non-interpretation time". Masland et al.'s (2010: 741–742) review is equally positive, underlining the advantages of RI (by telephone and video link) compared with F2FI, especially in terms of access, efficiency, quality of care and increased privacy. However, Masland et al. (*ibid.*) stress that for RI to be effective, specific provider and staff training in RI is essential. In most of the studies, the interpreters themselves also assessed RI as acceptable, while nevertheless generally preferring F2FI (Hornberger et al., 1996; Locatis et al., 2010, 2011; Paras et al., 2002). Among the RI methods, interpreters tended to prefer VI to TI, stating that seeing both the patient and the healthcare provider was extremely important to them (Paras et al., 2002).

However positive the overall results may seem, including such a wide range of factors (F2FI vs. RI; trained vs. informal interpreters; interpreter-mediated vs. non-mediated healthcare service) obscures the relative influence of each single feature, especially of the remote factors. Only five of the studies exclusively used trained interpreters to compare F2FI, TI and VI (Jones et al., 2003; Locatis et al., 2011; Paras, 2002; Price Leemann et al., 2012; Saint-Louis et al., 2003). Moreover, some of the research projects lacked a direct comparison between RI and F2FI. For example, in the study by Cunningham et al. (2008), none of the patients surveyed about their satisfaction with telephone interpreters had experience with interpreting, whether by means of F2FI or RI. Their high satisfaction with TI seemed therefore to have been the result of being happy to have an interpreter in the first place, while the results disclosed little about the remote factor. The same goes for Lee et al. (2002), whose study examined satisfaction with (professional) telephone interpreters compared to face-to-face interpreting by family members or friends.

With such a large variety of research designs and variables tested, even within one research discipline, it is hard to generalize the results of these studies. To put the positive results further into perspective, a few other critical notes must be taken into account, for example, the impact of the interpreting method. Some of the experiments involved simultaneous interpreting, whereas others used consecutive interpreting. For the simultaneous mode, the interpreters received specific training (Gany et al., 2007a; Hornberger et al., 1996; Saint-Louis et al., 2003), which may have influenced the positive results. Moreover, the use of simultaneous interpreting in healthcare settings seems rather unrealistic for the moment, given its more complex technological requirements that necessitate separate audio channels to avoid acoustic overlap when two spoken languages are involved (Pöchhacker, 2015: 308).

Furthermore, in the medical studies on RI, technological issues and their impact on the communication process are not frequently addressed. Only a few studies (Locatis et al., 2010, 2011) provide technical specifications of the videoconferencing appliances that were used, survey participant satisfaction with sound and visual quality in RI (Jones et al., 2003) or describe practical problems with technology and call for training and protocols on RI equipment use (Saint-Louis et al., 2003: 52). However, since most of the studies lack technical specifications, it is difficult to assess the impact of the technological factors. In the study by Garcia et al. (2004) on TI, for example, it is not clear how many patients used a dual headset phone or a standard telephone. Yet, this is important information, since the use of a standard telephone has been proven to diminish satisfaction with TI, because the patient and the healthcare provider must pass a single headset back and forth (Cunningham et al., 2008).

Since the medical studies often weigh costs and benefits against each other, a relevant research issue is the impact of the interpreting method and mode on consultation length (Fagan et al., 2003; Gany et al., 2007a; Jones et al., 2003; Locatis, 2010). Here again, a generalization of the results concerning consultation length is impossible, given the different methods (TI and VI) and modes (consecutive and simultaneous) that were used in each study. For example, Hornberger et al. (1996: 852) implemented an experiment comparing TI and F2FI and concluded that the average RI visit duration was more or less equal to the F2FI visit length. This observation was most likely related to the simultaneous mode in which the RI was delivered. In the study by Gany et al. (2007a: 321) on the impact of medical interpretation methods on duration and errors, it was found that RI conducted in the simultaneous mode was almost twice as fast as consecutive RI.

Studies based only on consecutive interpreting yielded more contradictory results concerning average consultation duration. In the study by Fagan et al. (2003), telephone and "patient-supplied" interpreters (i.e. informal interpreters) were associated with longer visit times compared with professional in-person hospital interpreters. By contrast, the research by Jones et al. (2003) concluded that mean consultation times were highest in VI and shortest in TI. Locatis et al. (2010) also observed that video set-up takes more time, rendering the waiting times longer compared to F2FI, while TI took the least time. The shorter duration of the TI consultations was explained by the fact that TI is an "outside service" in most of the hospitals, involving additional expenses, which may persuade providers to "adopt time-saving approaches" (*ibid.*). Moreover, there are fewer opportunities for increased side-talk between the interpreter and the healthcare provider in TI or for asking questions after the consultation, compared with F2FI (*ibid.*).

We can conclude from the medical studies on RI that the interpreting methods (F2FI versus RI) mostly affect the perception of the quality of the encounter. Obviously, assessments based on users' perceptions are a good indicator of user satisfaction, but they have the disadvantage of being subjective. Previous subjective assessment of interpreting quality in interpreting studies has indicated that interpreting clients are not necessarily in a position to assess an interpreter's performance (Shlesinger, 2007) and that client expectations tend to be less rigorous than interpreters' expectations (Braun, 2013). Moreover, in some of the experiments (Locatis et al., 2010), the patients participating were exposed to only one of the interpreting methods, whereas the healthcare providers and interpreters used all three methods, which may have made the healthcare providers and interpreters more sensitive to some specific limitations of the RI methods. As Price Leemann et al. (2012: 227) point out, interpreters, as opposed to patients, are "insiders" to the medical system and may therefore also be "more willing than patients to be openly critical of modalities that do not work well".

Furthermore, in some of the studies (Cunningham et al., 2008; Gany et al., 2007a, 2007b; García et al., 2004; Wofford et al., 2012), the interpreters themselves were not surveyed on their perceptions. Strangely enough, in the study by Wofford et al. (2012), the first keyword accompanying the abstract is "interpreter perspective", whereas the interpreter perceptions were in fact not included in the examination.

What is most striking about the medical studies, for researchers examining RI from an interpreting studies perspective, is the missed opportunity of evaluating the communication process and the interpreting performance itself in the data collected by these medical studies on RI. Only two of the studies actually assess the quality of the communication itself: Hornberger et al. (1996) and Gany et al. (2007a). These are also the only studies that integrate literature on translation, interpreting, and linguistics, such as Altman (1994), Barik (1994), Bugel-Shunra (2000), Kussmaul (1995) and MacCulloch (2001).

Hornberger et al. (1996) assessed the effects of remote simultaneous interpreting by telephone and face-to-face consecutive interpreting on the amount of information exchanged, the accuracy of the interpretation and users' preferences between the two interpreting methods. Patients were randomly assigned to one of the methods. Subsequently, the encounters were tape-recorded and coded. In a first session, the amount and type of information in the exchanges between the patient and the physician involved were coded ("questions", "instructions" – only by the physician –, "explanations" and "requests for clarity"); in a second session, the accuracy of the interpreting was coded ("addition", "omission" or "substitution") (*ibid.*: 849). The results regarding the quality of the communication were very much in favour of the RI methods. In the RI sessions, more utterances were observed, as well as fewer inaccuracies (*ibid.*: 852). Considered from the perspective of interpreting studies, the linguistic analysis was quite limited, since the consultations were studied only at a text level and did not take into account the interaction that shapes the content. Moreover, the remote simultaneous interpreters had received specific instructions to ask for clarification in case of uncertainty about meaning (*ibid.*: 848), whereas there was no mention of this to the face-to-face consecutive interpreters. This may have influenced the more positive results as well. The same goes for the instructions telling the remote interpreters to speak in the first person, whereas the face-to-face interpreters received no such instructions and used the third person to refer to the primary participants (*ibid.*). Hornberger et al. (1996: 852) remarked that simultaneous interpretation requires interpreters to "use the first-person tense and accurately interpret each phrase" to abide by the AIIC code of conduct, yet they failed to recognize that this is just as true for consecutive interpreters, who also follow their professional codes. The fact that only the RI-method interpreter adopted the first-person perspective (saying "I" when interpreting for any of the primary participants) may have also contributed to the increased rapport reported by the physician from the RI-method session. In medical encounters, rapport refers to the relationship between the healthcare provider and the patient, which consists of trust and mutual responsiveness and fosters the therapeutic process (Farlex, 2012).

Gany et al. (2007a: 320) also looked at accuracy (as well as speed) and added a medical dimension to Barik's 1994 error analysis by distinguishing between linguistic and medical errors, which they defined as "meaningful linguistic errors with medical information". Scripted clinical encounters were audiotaped, transcribed and coded to measure the impact of various interpreting methods on interpreting speed and errors. These methods consisted of remote simultaneous, remote consecutive, face-to-face consecutive and face-to-face ad hoc (i.e. untrained) interpreters. A linguistic error was considered a medical error if the language made reference to something that was medically related, according to a scale of clinical significance ranging from clinically insignificant to mildly, moderately and highly clinically significant to potentially life-threatening (*ibid.*: 320). The study also concluded that remote simultaneous interpreting was the most accurate interpreting method.

Other medical studies have assessed the "efficacy" of the communication. For example, Crossman et al. (2010) verified concordance between caregivers' descriptions of a patient's diagnosis and the physician's stated discharge diagnosis between F2FI and TI, finding no significant differences. Price Leemann et al. (2012) investigated the adequacy of RI methods for specific communication needs and certain scenarios in healthcare situations as perceived by professional interpreters, which led to the identification of situations in which F2FI, TI or VI were most suited. They concluded that, from the interpreter's perspective, TI was satisfactory for the exchange of information, but less so for interpersonal aspects of communication, for which VI was better suited (*ibid.*: 226). According to the same research, effective communication in clinical encounters depends on "the exchange of accurate information", "interpersonal skills that foster understanding of patients' social or cultural backgrounds" and "the development of patient–clinician rapport" (*ibid.*). Rapport was particularly affected in RI (both in TI and VI), according to the interpreters in the study by Price Leemann et al. (*ibid.*: 229).

However, as far as rapport between patient and care provider is concerned, other medical studies have generated opposing results depending on the participants. The aforementioned study by Hornberger et al. (1996: 854) found that healthcare providers using remote simultaneous interpretation by telephone could develop "even greater rapport than is achievable with existing language services" compared with consecutive F2FI. In the study by Saint-Louis et al. (2003: 51), who compared VI to TI and consecutive F2FI, nearly all interpreters commented that they felt that the "use of the remote interpreting methods brought the patient and provider closer together since the interpreter was not physically present". Interview data analysed by Jones et al. (2003: 55) show that more patients felt shy and nervous in F2FI, which, according to the researchers, suggests that for some patients, the interpreter's social presence with the patient and the doctor may make patients uncomfortable.

Interestingly, the medical study by Saint-Louis et al. (2003: 48) is the only study to mention the impact of the remote conditions on the role of the interpreter. It emphasizes the lack of access to complete visual information on the part of the interpreter in settings of video remote interpreting, that is, when the doctor and patient are together and the interpreter is in a separate location. Moreover, according to the same study, the role of the interpreter differs in RI compared with F2FI. When RI methods were used, the healthcare providers actually missed the opportunity to talk privately with the interpreter and receive extra information about cultural issues and other similar input (*ibid.*: 52).

What is most obvious after reviewing the medical studies, is that they, as opposed to research in interpreting studies, attempt to paint a picture of the interpreter-mediated clinical visit as a whole, with the interpreter as only one of many factors being researched. However, the idea of comparing the three different interpreting methods (F2FI, TI and VI) appears to be a useful way to assess the individual peculiarities of each method. If the analysis of participants' perceptions and preferences were complemented by an analysis of the quality of the interpreted communication, as is proposed in this work, this type of comparative research could generate broader insights into the remote conditions' impact on the quality of interpreter-mediated communication.

2.2.2 Interpreting studies

Research in RI within interpreting studies often uses perspectives from the humanities – such as sociology, communication studies and pragmatics – and is, therefore, often more or less multidisciplinary. These studies mostly set out to identify and investigate potential difficulties specific to interpreter-mediated remote communication. With the exception of the report from a more recent project in interpreting studies (Shift in Orality, <www.shiftinorality.eu>), which brings together research on both telephone interpreting (TI) and video interpreting (VI) and has resulted in the *Handbook of Remote Interpreting* (Amato et al., 2018), most of the academic research examines either TI or VI. I will first look into the research on TI and will then discuss the outcomes from studies on VI). Again, this overview is by no means exhaustive and focuses on the studies that are most relevant to the current research objectives.

Telephone interpreting

As explained in Section 1.2, telephone interpreting (TI) refers to situations in which the interpreter works over the telephone, either at the same location as one of the interlocutors (teleconference interpreting; TCI) or at a separate location (telephone remote interpreting; TRI). The majority of the studies discussed below examined the latter variant. TI is usually performed in the consecutive mode, although a "teleconference bridge" would allow for simultaneous interpreting (O'Hagan, 1996: 77). The research on TI is relatively scarce and shows a scattered field, as Ozolins (2011: 41) points out in his overview of research and research needs on the subject of TI:

> Such a research history – with different authors putting quite different emphasis on various aspects of TI (first/third person; the question of visuals; modes of TI setup; remuneration; discourse; commitment) – rather than giving us a good overall picture of TI, has resulted in no study being replicated and potential hypotheses raised never being tested in other studies.

The themes examined by empirical studies in this field (Amato et al., 2018; Castagnoli & Niemants, 2018; Fernández-Pérez, 2017; Ko, 2006; Lee, 2007; Oviatt & Cohen, 1992; Rosenberg, 2007; Wadensjö, 1999; Wang, 2018; Wang & Fang, 2019) vary greatly indeed. Topics range from linguistic, cognitive and interactional issues and interpreters' capacity to adapt to new communicative situations, to the remote situation's impact on interpreter working conditions, including remuneration. Some studies focus on interpreters' perceptions of TI, such as Wang (2018), who conducted a large survey to analyse interpreters' opinions on the quality and suitability of TI, whereas other studies explore specific features of telephone interpreting (Fernández-Pérez, 2017; Spinolo et al., 2018b). Fernández-Pérez's (2017) summary of specific TI features is quite representative of the different themes discussed in TI research. She mentions the physical absence of the interpreter, the lack of visual access and "contextualization cues" (Gumperz, 1982), as well as the immediacy with which users have access to the interpreter (Fernández-Pérez, 2017). According to Amato and Spinolo's (2018: 8) review of TI research, the lack of visual access complicates the turn-taking organization, which creates communicative uncertainty among TI users. Amato and Spinolo (*ibid.*) also put forward technological issues in TI, such as bad sound quality, as well as practical problems, for example, the enormous variety of topics that telephone interpreters have to deal with. However, the latter issue does not seem to be unique to TI, but rather to the profession of community interpreting in general. In a more recent publication based on the corpus collected by the project "Shift in Orality" mentioned in the introduction to this section, Iglesias-Fernández and Russo (2020) propose a multidisciplinary methodological approach in studying TI as a social activity, as technologized interaction and as talk, including the analysis of prosody in steering the interaction. Their idea of integrating various approaches in exposing discursive mechanisms underlying TI, aims to enhance current interpreter training.

The first important empirical study on TI was conducted by Oviatt and Cohen (1992: 277), who compared "three-person interpreted telephone dialogues", which included a professional telephone interpreter, with "two-person non-interpreted calls", in order to examine "the unique discourse and performance characteristics of interpreted telephone speech during service-oriented exchanges". The study's main conclusions were that in interpreter-mediated telephone conversations, the interpreter has a pivotal role in regulating turn-taking and actively managing the conversation. Telephone interpreters used "I" and "me" self-referentially, and the third-person pronoun to refer to the parties they interpreted for, which is also referred to as "reported speech" (Bot, 2005), instead of maintaining the speaker's perspective by using the first person ("direct speech"). The latter is considered the professional norm in dialogue interpreting (*ibid.*). According to Oviatt and Cohen (1992: 286), the use of reported speech proved that the interpreters were actively involved in the coordination of the conversations. In so doing, they avoided potential miscommunication caused by the lack of visual input. In the same study, another interactional aspect, overlapping speech, was hypothesized to occur more often in three-way interpreter-mediated telephone conversations. However, this did not turn out to be the case in the experiments (*ibid.*: 288). The interpreter-mediated calls did show a higher rate of "confirmation language" (*ibid.*), a synonym for meta communication. This consisted of requests for information, listener backchannels such as "hm" and "okay", "yes" and "sure", and confirmations, that is, the repetition of, for example, numbers and letters (*ibid.*: 283–284). These utterances accounted for nearly one third of the total of spoken words in TI, compared to less than a quarter of the spoken words during non-mediated telephone conversations. According to

O'Hagan and Ashworth (2002: 103), increased explicit confirmation language can be a way to compensate for the lack of nonverbal cues. Despite these compensations, in the study by Oviatt and Cohen (1992: 287) miscommunication was higher in TI than in the non-mediated telephone calls under investigation.

In line with Oviatt and Cohen (1992), Wadensjö (1999: 247) argues in her descriptive study comparing participants' behaviour in TI and F2FI during police interviews that, in TI, the interpreter makes an additional effort to "coordinate and synchronize the interaction". Wadensjö (*ibid.*) found that F2FI, compared with TI, was more fluent and she also observed differences in the average length of the participants' "turns at talk" and in "patterns of overlapping speech". In TI, the turns of the interpreter were longer than in F2FI, reducing the "time slots" available for the primary participants (*ibid.*: 256–257). As far as overlapping speech is concerned, Wadensjö (*ibid.*: 257) cites Tannen (1984: 146) to argue that, in ordinary conversation, overlap of talk occurs naturally and is called "cooperative overlap" when it is used as a way for an interlocutor to communicate positive involvement. In the F2FI encounter, Wadensjö (*ibid.*) noticed that overlaps occurred frequently, since the interpreter started her renditions often before the primary speakers' turns were finished completely. According to the scholar (*ibid.*: 260) these early starts were "a matter of timing" and did not happen "just at any moment, but in micro-pauses" or, citing Schegloff (1996: 97), in "transition spaces". In TI, the moments of transition occurring between participants' turns were generally longer in duration, which was considered a way to avoid overlapping speech, but also led to confusion about who was to speak next in TI (Wadensjö, 1999). According to Wadensjö (*ibid.*: 261), moments of "feedback", that is, utterances with the purpose of checking or confirming whether a message has been understood – called "confirmation language" by Oviatt and Cohen (1992) –, as well as short, vocalized utterances expressing the listener's involvement in the communication, often occur during or as a result of overlaps. In TI, there was less feedback, as a result of which, the speech was "altogether less fluent", compared with F2FI (Wadensjö, 1999: 264).

Both the studies by Wadensjö (1999) and Oviatt and Cohen (1992) were criticized by Rosenberg (2007) because of the small samples of data.

Moreover, according to the latter (*ibid*.: 67), they are based on the assumption that all TI calls are basically similar, an idea that the scholar challenges. Rosenberg (2007: 65) collected authentic TI data over a two-year period and examined their features in three distinct communication configurations of consecutive TI: (1) three-way telephone calls with all three parties in different locations, (2) F2FI conversations interpreted by a telephone remote interpreter using speakerphones and (3) F2FI conversations interpreted by a telephone remote interpreter, with the participants passing the telephone back and forth. The findings of this study indicate that the complexity of TI was not so much due to inherent linguistic differences between TI and F2FI, but was instead the result of the interpreter's "expanding access". That means that telephone interpreters must be available to a larger and more heterogeneous population (as opposed to the more "intimate" work settings in F2FI) and, as such, face a large variety in assignments, stretching their capacities to the limit (*ibid*.: 74–75). Moreover, as Rosenberg (*ibid*.: 75) argues, the physical distance and lack of a shared frame of reference between the geographically separated interlocutors in TI renders the interpreting task more complex. In addition, the obvious difference between F2FI and TI, that is, the lack of visual contact, can be turned into an advantage of TI because of the increased privacy and lesser degree of distraction for the interpreter (*ibid*.). Based on his own experience as an interpreter, Rosenberg (*ibid*.: 67) considered the poor sound quality associated with TI to simply be a part of the interpreter's generally "noisy working environment". As for the use of reported speech, like Oviatt and Cohen (1992), Rosenberg (2007: 74) observed that interpreters and primary speakers predominantly used reported speech in TI. Reported speech was observed in 85 per cent of the three-way and speakerphone TI conversations, and in 100 per cent of the cases of TI by passing the telephone. The large differences in efficacy and accuracy of the interpretation between the three configurations (of which "passing of the telephone" turned out to be the most problematic), showed that the types of devices used influenced interpreting performance. However, since Rosenberg's study lacks benchmarking with F2FI interpreter-mediated communication, not all issues reported were necessarily specifically related to TI. Moreover, as put forward earlier in this section, it could be argued that the diversity of the assignments, which, according to Rosenberg (2007), complicates the work of telephone interpreters, may not be exclusive to TI, but a daily reality for most freelance community interpreters, whose work may take them into various domains in the same day (Tebble, 2012).

The influence of the technical conditions on interpreting performance is also advanced by Ko (2006), who set up an experiment involving six interpreters with no previous experience in TI. The interpreters carried out simulated TI calls in eight sessions over four weeks, during which data were collected from the participants' diaries and by means of questionnaires and interviews. In line with Rosenberg (2007), Ko (2006: 332) established that the use of different types of equipment had different effects on the interpreters' comfort levels. Hands-free telephone devices, such as mobile phones with headphones and speakerphones were considered more comfortable by the interpreters, because they did not to have to hold a phone or a receiver while taking notes. The interpreters using conventional devices that did not allow for hands-free calling were reported to feel most uncomfortable with TI and also showed a shorter concentration span. As soon as they switched to the hands-free devices, the problems of discomfort were not reported again (*ibid*.: 332). After a period of interpreting practice, the interpreters were able to overcome problems of fatigue associated with working in TI and their concentration span increased. Moreover, the lack of visual access became less problematic as the experience with TI increased (*ibid*.: 333–334).

Technical issues in TI were also examined by Lee (2007), who surveyed twenty Korean telephone interpreters. Examples of such technical problems were bad sound quality, lack of a three-way connection and disconnection. Apart from these issues, lack of physical contact and visual information were mentioned as major challenges of TI, which, according to Lee (*ibid*.: 240–241), largely outweighed aspects that were mentioned as positive, such as enhanced neutrality and concentration, and the convenience of working from home. Although the emphasis of Lee's (*ibid*.) study is mostly on working conditions, some interactional issues were also touched upon, such as the organization of the dialogue and reported speech. Based on her survey data, the author concluded that most telephone interpreters found they actively facilitated and managed the conversation. Interestingly, the ways in which the interpreters perceived their roles depended on their accreditation level. Significant differences were observed between fully accredited and partly accredited interpreters. The latter group stated that they were actively involved in facilitating and managing the conversation, whereas in the former group, only less than half of the interpreters indicated that they facilitated phone conversations. Most of them replied they "just interpreted" (*ibid*.: 245). According to Lee (*ibid*.), fully certified interpreters may be more conscious of their roles an interpreter. As far as reported speech is concerned, Lee (*ibid*.: 246) found that

> all of [the interpreters] stated that they were aware of "first-person interpreting", but not all of them practiced it, and only 40% invariably used the first person. 15% [...] interpreted in the third person, and 45% [...] mixed first and third person. Telephone interpreters stated that they tended to interpret in the third person more often over the phone than face-to-face. Some intentionally used third-person interpreting to avoid misunderstanding and to make clear who said what.

Almost all of the interpreters using the first person maintained that they found it difficult to do so in TI and admitted that they occasionally needed to intervene by adding explicitly "I, the interpreter" when the communication did not run smoothly (*ibid*.: 247) or by mixing the use of the first and third person to avoid confusion. Lee (*ibid*.) considered this proof of active conversation management by interpreters in TI.

The increased role of telephone interpreters in facilitating the communication is confirmed by Wang (2018) in her survey analysing interpreters' perceptions of quality and suitability of TI. A more recent study by Wang and Fang (2019) is one of the few studies comparing accuracy in TI and F2FI. The scholars created a "meaning-unit" quality assessment framework for micro-analyses in order to explain the nature of accurate interpretations and of problematic cases. Scenarios derived from authentic social service settings encounters were simulated in F2FI and TI. After completing the simulations, the (experienced) interpreter engaged in a short, semi-structured interview. The results of the data analyses indicate that the interpreter participating in the simulations performed equally well in both F2FI and TI in terms of accuracy of the interpretation, although the number of "unjustifiable" omissions was marginally higher in TI (*ibid*.: 45). Some of these omissions were the result of interpreting difficulties in the source text, poor sound quality, cognitive overload and the fact that the interpreter did not interrupt the primary speakers during longer turns (*ibid*.: 57). In TI, the interaction management was somewhat increased, as expressed by a (slightly) higher number of strategic additions. Although the interactional context was taken into account in the microanalyses of the simulations, only voice-recordings were done. Moreover, since only one interpreter participated in three different scenarios, the results cannot be generalized.

Summarizing the research on TI, we can conclude that, despite disparities in methodology and design in this research field, the findings show similarities with respect to technical and interactional issues. The research indicates that the technical circumstances in which TI takes place influence the perception of convenience and quality of the TI performance. In addition, telephone interpreters are more actively involved in the coordination of the conversation, by being more explicit when referring to themselves and to the primary participants and by facilitating dialogue. They do so by intervening to avoid miscommunication and overlapping talk. However, since only few studies provided a direct comparison between TI and F2FI, it cannot be established to which degree the observed issues were specific to the TI conditions. Moreover, the studies predominantly investigate the interpreters' perceptions of TI, without a more objective assessment of the quality or accuracy of the performance, with the exception of Wang and Fang (2019). Even when more objective methods were used (Rosenberg, 2007), the lack of comparison with the F2FI interpreting method makes it difficult to put the findings into perspective. In addition, the research often focuses on interpreters' perceptions and neglects the perception of the other users of TI services (such as clients) involved in the interpreting process. Therefore, the research on TI clearly shows a need for methods combining the assessment of the interpreting process and performance from the point of view of the different parties involved, in direct comparison to F2FI. Such a comparison, as performed in the current research, is useful to establish to which degree certain communication features and issues are specific to each particular interpreting method. In addition, the investigation of accuracy in TI is clearly a knowledge gap in interpreting studies that I attempt to bridge with this work.

Video interpreting

Video interpreting refers to different configurations of RI by means of video link, most often carried out in the consecutive mode, with the exception of Pöchhacker (2014). As we saw in Section 1.2, there are different configurations of VI. Firstly, in VCI (videoconference interpreting), the communication takes place in two different video-linked locations, with the interpreter physically present with one of the parties. Secondly, in VRI (video remote interpreting), the primary participants are in the same location, but the interpreter works from a separate location (Braun & Taylor, 2012a: 39–41). A third constellation that has become more common since the introduction of lockdown measures due to the outbreak of COVID-19 is so-called "three-way" VI, in which all participants are in different locations.

Compared to the research on TI, the research on VI is more often (although not always) benchmarked against F2FI. Moreover, the research angle of VI studies appears to be larger and more holistic. Although the interpreter's performance is the central theme, the actions and reactions of the other parties involved in the dialogue interpreting situation are also scrutinized, as well as the communicative process, the technical circumstances, the context and the visibility of the interpreter. While early research focused on business interpreting (Braun, 2001, 2003, 2004; Braun & Kohn, 2001), the largest projects on VI were carried out in the context of legal interpreting. More recently, research findings in VI carried out in different dialogue interpreting settings were brought together in the *Handbook of Remote Interpreting* (Amato et al., 2018). As mentioned earlier, this collection of research on TI and VI presents an overview of much-addressed issues in RI. It also describes basic requirements for successful RI and provides teaching materials specifically designed for training remote interpreters. As far as VI is concerned, the handbook puts forward that, in the different types of RI, important nonverbal cues that users are familiar with in F2FI are less effective due to the "spatial, technical and sensory constraints that these [RI] channels inevitably bring with them" (Spinolo et al., 2018b: 19). The handbook also draws attention to interactional issues that are specific to VI or are magnified by this interpreting method (Davitti & Braun, 2018: 119) and emphasizes that the variations in research findings in different interpreting contexts imply that a one-size-fits-all approach in the application of RI services is "unlikely to work" (Braun & Davitti, 2018: 114). Although the interactional character of remote dialogue interpreting has been investigated thoroughly, only few studies have carried out micro-analytical investigations highlighting multimodal aspects, such as Davitti (2018), Licoppe and Vernier (2013), Licoppe and Veyrier (2017) and Davitti and Braun (2020).

In the following sections, research on VI in specific contexts is discussed in more detail. We will discuss the fields of business interpreting, legal interpreting, healthcare interpreting and other settings of dialogue interpreting. The section concludes with a brief summary of the results of research on VI carried out in different sign language interpreting contexts.

BUSINESS INTERPRETING

In interpreting studies, Braun (2001, 2003, 2004) and Braun and Kohn (2001) were among the first researchers to study VI. In her studies on video-mediated interpreting, Braun extensively discusses research on monolingual video-mediated communication (Anderson et al., 1997; O'Connaill et al., 1997; Olson et al., 1997; O'Malley et al., 1996; Sellen, 1995; Sellen & Harper, 1997; Short et al., 1976; Tang & Isaacs, 1993) to identify fundamental issues relevant to VI. Among these issues are the effects of geographical separation, technical mediation and the availability of visual information on users' perceptions of the communication and on their communicative behaviour. Questions raised in this research include whether video-mediated communication can replicate the conversational processes in F2FI communication and what effects video-mediation has on the internal organization of communication processes. The research also looked into the process of users' familiarization with new communication channels, the efficiency of video-mediation, users' acceptance, and optimization of videoconferencing are applied to VI (Braun, 2004). Whereas in video-mediated monolingual communication, the separation in geographical space between the participants appears to cause social distance, in VI, the distance imposed by the different languages and cultures must additionally be taken into account, as well as the potential impact of interactional problems (*ibid.*: 97).

Braun (2004) also analysed the specific interactional aspects of face-to-face dialogue interpreting to establish how interpreter-mediated communication differs from non-mediated communication. Based on her analysis of the interactional characteristics of face-to-face dialogue interpreting (turn-taking, pauses, overlapping speech, interruptions and backchannelling), Braun's (*ibid.*) experiments showed how these interactional features were affected in VI. For example, turn-taking followed a different pattern in VI than in F2FI. Moreover, floor holding, taking over of the floor, intended and unintended pauses, as well as competitive and non-competitive overlapping speech, all functioned differently in the experiments in VI compared with F2FI. Because of the difference in timing that resulted from the delay of sound and image, pauses, interruptions and backchannelling were often not perceived the way they were intended. The additional difficulties that occurred when the interpreting took place under technically mediated audiovisual conditions were further reinforced when users were not familiar with this medium (*ibid.*: 85). However, as Braun (2007, 2013) emphasized in her later studies on VI, communication must be considered a strategic process of optimization. Consequently, despite interactional and cognitive problems in VI that affect message content, speech comprehension and speech production, participants adapt their conversational behaviour in order to achieve their communicative goals. According to Braun (2004: 164–166), participants do this by using monitoring and supporting strategies to optimize communication by continually verifying comprehension and production results through both verbal and nonverbal signals. In her opinion, these signals differed in VI compared with F2FI.

LEGAL INTERPRETING

As far as legal interpreting is concerned, the use of videoconference technology is promoted by the European e-Justice initiative and is increasingly considered a potential solution for gaining cost-efficiency and timely access to qualified legal interpreters (Braun & Taylor, 2012a). Therefore, it is not surprising that the largest research projects on VI were carried out in the legal context. The projects AVIDICUS 1, 2, and 3 (2008–2016)[3] and DUTT (Developing the Use of Technical Tools for Cross-Border Resettlement, 2011–2013)[4] were both supported by the Criminal Justice Programme of the European Commission. AVIDICUS 1 and 2 evaluated the viability and quality of video-based interpreting in criminal proceedings with a focus on communication. The quality of the interpreters' VI performance in criminal proceedings was investigated, involving partners in several European countries and external experts in videoconference technology, communication, legal interpreting and training. The outcomes of the projects were collected as chapters in the work *Videoconference and Remote Interpreting in Criminal Proceedings*, edited by Braun and Taylor (2012a). This was the first study on VI in legal settings involving multiple countries and different VI configurations, that is, VRI and VCI (Braun, 2018). Central to this project were a series of empirical studies consisting of experiments involving police interviews (Balogh & Hertog, 2012). These experiments compared the quality of the different audiovisual VI constellations (VCI and VRI) with F2FI. As in Braun and Taylor's (2012b) prior research, much attention is paid to changes in interactional dynamics in interpreter-mediated remote communication and to the cognitive complexity of interpreting, which is further reinforced by the technological mediation. The experiments were analysed using assessment categories – which included language-based as well as nonverbal and "audiovisual" categories – that were coded by a team of raters and then quantified in order to analyse interpreting quality in VCI and VRI in comparison with F2FI. The expectation was that the number of problems would be higher in VI than in F2FI in all of the categories. This was confirmed by the analysis of most of the individual series of simulations, albeit to various degrees (*ibid.*: 92). For example, in the simulations studied by Balogh and Hertog (2012), few quality differences were observed across the VI configurations and F2FI. In VI, a stronger correlation was observed overall between interactional categories (such

---

3   <http://wp.videoconference-interpreting.net>.
4   <https://www.cep-probation.org/projects/developing-the-use-of-technical-tools-in-cross-border-resettlement-dutt>.

as turn-taking problems) and accuracy issues, especially omissions, when compared with F2FI (Braun & Taylor, 2012b). The various studies within the project also put forward that the recurrence of overlapping speech and its consequences suggests that avoiding and managing overlapping speech is an important issue for VI guidelines and training (*ibid.*: 94). Moreover, the results of the experiments confirmed earlier findings from research on RI in conference settings concerning fatigue, which was considered the likeliest reason for the steeper increase of problems in VI halfway through the sessions (*ibid.*: 95). Moreover, the average speech rate was observed to be lower in VI, which was considered a possible explanation for the longer average duration of the VI sessions. However, as Braun & Taylor (*ibid.*: 96) argue:

> A more detailed qualitative analysis of the data shows that the video-based sessions also required what Olson, Olson & Meader (1997, p. 170) called a greater "process overhead", for example, to coordinate the communication or to resolve comprehension problems. This would explain why all groups of participants used a slightly higher number of words in the video-mediated sessions.

Braun and Taylor (*ibid.*: 93) conclude that, because of the specific requirements of legal interpreting, the issues identified in their study put constraints on the use of VI in criminal proceedings. These issues include differences in length, which suggests that the VI sessions were overall less efficient than F2FI (*ibid.*: 96). In addition, as the authors argue, problems with overlapping speech may jeopardize rapport-building (*ibid.*: 97). As it turned out, familiar interpreting strategies such as the use of visual signs to control the floor were often not effective in VI, whereas alternative strategies, such as verbal intervention, were likely to disrupt the communication flow and create uncertainty among the participants.

The second part of the project, AVIDICUS 2, proved that specific training for VI purposes did have a beneficial effect on communication management. After all participants had undergone specific training on VI, the number of turn-taking problems and overlaps in VI diminished (*ibid.*: 316).

Lastly, AVIDICUS 3 turned to the design and implementation of bilingual VI solutions across legal institutions in 12 EU-member states.

The AVIDICUS projects also led to the development of guidelines for video-link use in legal settings, as well as training modules and a handbook (*Handbook of Bilingual Videoconferencing*[5]). Although the research results were very mixed, they showed that

> the complexities of interpreter-mediated communication and bilingual videoconferencing are generally under-estimated by legal and institutional stakeholders, and that they need to gain a more comprehensive understanding of the specific requirements that arise from the combination of VC and interpreter-mediated communication in legal settings. (Avidicus 3 [2014–2016], Aims and outcomes[6])

The outcomes of another large project reported by Braun and Taylor (2013), DUTT, suggest more positive conclusions. The project investigated the benefits and challenges of videoconference technology to support cross-border communication in relation to cross-border resettlement procedures. The research involved simulations representing different linguistic configurations, including the use of a second language, a lingua franca and communication through an interpreter (*ibid.*: 1). The analysis of the problems observed indicates that VC communication (with and without an interpreter) was a useful addition to the communication tools available for cross-border communication (alongside telephone and email), provided that a number of technical – and other – conditions were met. Most of the problems identified seemed to be related to a lack of participant experience, which can be remedied when basic guidelines are followed (*ibid.*: 47). Also, some clear advantages of VI were observed, compared with TI. VI allowed for small-group communication and reduced the number of individual one-to-one conversations held via telephone. Moreover, it permitted visual assessment of offenders and allowed participants to use visual cues to check if their utterances had been understood, thus facilitating the detection of comprehension problems. In addition, VI led to smoother turn-taking, as the interpreters were able to indicate which interlocutor they were interpreting for using visual

---

5 <http://www.videoconference-interpreting.net/wp-content/uploads/2016/08/AVIDICUS3_Handbook_Bilingual_Videoconferencing.pdf>.
6 <http://wp.videoconference-interpreting.net/?page_id=154>.

signs (*ibid*.: 48). The study shows that the benefits of VC technology are related to the achievement of the specific goals of legal communication, that is, fairness of justice and mutual trust, which is possible when VI meets minimum standards and codes of best practice with regard to a range of parameters that are closely connected to each other:

> In the first place, the quality of the technology, together with the audiovisual environment, has an impact on participant interaction and mutual perception, laying the foundation for inter alia role clarity. Following on from this, the clarity of participant roles and of procedures is an important prerequisite for ensuring that the information exchanged is appropriate and relevant for the purpose. Problems with roles and procedures, of course, also create problems with the interaction. (*ibid*.: 50)

Another, more recent study by Braun (2018) investigating interpreters' perceptions of VI in legal settings in the UK reported mostly negative interpreter experiences with this type of RI. This was mostly due to the inadequate local VI conditions and the fact that the interpreters had not been involved in the technical set-up, which could have contributed to a more adequate technological environment (*ibid*.: 416).

In the legal field (prison/court hearings), several other research projects were carried out by, amongst others, Fowler (2007). This scholar reported many problems, such as technical issues (insufficient auditory signals), a lack of training of interpreters for the specific demands of VI and a lack of visual clues as a result of failure to track the participants by camera. As a result, Fowler (*ibid*.: 17) advised against using interpreters in prison video-link hearings.

Two further studies in the legal context by Licoppe and Vernier (2013) and Licoppe and Veyrier (2017) looked specifically into video interpreting in the courtroom. Licoppe and Vernier (2013) adopted a video-ethnographic and conversation analytic perspective to study the interaction during a pre-trial hearing between the participants in a "distributed" courtroom, with a remote defendant connected by video link from his prison location and the other participants (including the interpreter) together in the courtroom. The study discusses the implications of VCI with respect to the production of extended turns in a multilingual courtroom setting, taking into account multimodal aspects of this type of communication. It shows how, in VCI, the roles of participants in the courtroom differ from the usual ones in a "normal", co-present courtroom. This was related to the limited visual access of the participants and brought about "interactional asymmetries" (*ibid.*: 249). The second study by Licoppe and Veyrier (2017) also focusses primarily on the pragmatic impact of the visual ecology in the courtroom. It shows in which way the choices (by the judge) of how the interpreter was displayed on the screen (alone or together with one of the primary participants) impacted on the participation status of the interpreter.

Outside of Europe, several larger research projects in the legal context were carried out, for example, by Ellis (2004), who reviewed the use of VCI in refugee hearings in Canada to assess the impact of technology on the fairness and efficiency of the hearings by means of interviews, surveys and observations. Like in the DUTT project, the issue of building mutual trust came up and was considered difficult in VCI. Other problems mentioned by the participants included the lack of direct eye contact, the impersonal nature of VC, its negative impact on the interaction and technical problems. Other issues observed were the participants' inability to act informally off-the-record, additional stress and anxiety, and handling of documents. Ellis's (2004, Introduction, para. 15) main conclusion was that no final decision about the "appropriateness" of the use of VI in refugee hearings should be made without the investigation of further and more sophisticated trials. However, the research does not make entirely clear what exactly is understood by the term "appropriateness".

HEALTHCARE INTERPRETING

In the field of healthcare interpreting, a few empirical studies have been conducted on VI from the perspective of interpreting studies and humanities. The research resembles the medical studies on VI (as discussed in Section 3.1), in the sense that user satisfaction, measured by means of surveys and guided interviews with all the parties involved, is a central point of interest. Interestingly, the majority of these studies was conducted in Austria (Havelka, 2018; Korak, 2010; Koller & Pöchhacker, 2018; Pöchhacker, 2014).

Korak's (2010) study investigated whether or not interpreting via Skype was a viable alternative to F2FI (called "*in situ* interpreting") in healthcare.

The scholar collected data, based on real-life VRI sessions on Skype between doctors and patients in a hospital and remote interpreters working from their computer at home. The data were collected by means of questionnaires, guided interviews with doctors and interpreters, and replay sessions with the interpreters. During these sessions, the interpreters listened to the audio recordings of their performance and were invited to comment on these. Since only a small number of interpreters, using different language pairs, participated in the sessions, the data lack comparability, making it difficult to establish to what extent the problems observed in the research were related to the remote condition or the capacities of the individual interpreters and the local circumstances. The main research question, whether VI through Skype is "viable", was not fully answered, since no real definition of this concept of viability was provided. The study concludes that in a technical sense, VRI through Skype is possible, provided that a solid internet connection is used, as well as a computer with good processing capacities and fast random-access memory. Although the data can hardly be generalized, typical issues observed in previous VI research in other settings, such as feelings of alienation, reported speech, less coherent content and overlapping speech, were confirmed by this research.

Pöchhacker's (2014) research project on VRI involved experiments with simultaneous interpreting and consecutive interpreting conducted in an Austrian hospital. The project explored the "viability, acceptability and feasibility of VC-based simultaneous and consecutive interpreting" in authentic paediatric encounters, assessed from the perspective of patients, care providers and interpreters (*ibid*.: 310–312). Two experiments involved two different interpreter teams using VRI, one in consecutive and the other in simultaneous mode. The data consisted of semi-structured interviews, recordings and direct observations. The findings were rather in favour of the use of technology. However, whereas the dual VC system proved "fully satisfactory", the audio equipment caused problems (*ibid*.: 319). Although the test was not implemented as planned (i.e. with a direct comparison between the two modes, simultaneous and consecutive), the data generated indicated that simultaneous VRI was as functional and acceptable as consecutive VRI, especially among patients and interpreters (*ibid*.: 320).

Further positive findings from research on VI in healthcare settings were reported by Koller and Pöchhacker (2018), who investigated the experiences of a small group of young interpreters working for a VRI company specializing in healthcare settings. The interpreters perceived no major differences between VRI and F2FI and did not report any of the limitations of VRI described in previous studies. Moreover, the interpreters mentioned specific benefits from the remote conditions, such as feeling less pressure and distraction than at the hospital. However, as Koller and Pöchhacker (*ibid.*: 107) argue, the high levels of satisfaction of the interpreters may have been partly related to the working conditions in VI compared with F2FI, since the interpreters enjoyed working in teams in call centres, as opposed to working individually as freelance onsite interpreters.

Another Austrian study by Havelka (2018) reported on a pilot project involving five interpreters using VRI in a hospital setting, focussing mainly on their subjective assessment. The results of these data suggest that VRI showed numerous differences compared with F2FI interpreter-mediated interventions. These were especially related to feelings of alienation among the video remote interpreters – confirming results from research on remote conference interpreting (Moser-Mercer, 2005a, 2005b) – caused generally by the lack of contextual information in VRI. Furthermore, the interpreters reported that technical issues and the lack of interlocutor visibility, as well as a lack of preparation time in VRI, made the interpreting task more complex compared with F2FI (Havelka, 2018: 333).

A Belgian project by Verrept (2011) and Verrept et al. (2018) on remote intercultural healthcare mediation – called "Intercultural mediation through the internet" – was also based on real-life data. Its purpose was to make the services of intercultural mediators available at a larger scale in healthcare institutions in Belgium, by using a video link between intercultural mediators and healthcare providers.[7] After a first experiment in

---

[7] In Belgium, there is a strict differentiation between the tasks of "intercultural mediators" and "social interpreters" (literal translation from Dutch) in terms of neutrality and interventions. Social interpreters are community interpreters, who must abide by the strict rules of neutrality as provided in the Flemish code of conduct that stipulate, for example, that the interpreter has no right or duty to intervene to provide additional explanations to clients. By contrast, intercultural mediators, as the term implies, are allowed more freedom in their renditions, for example, to explain certain matters. See <https://www.health.belgium.be/en/health/taking-care-yourself/patient-related-themes/intercultural-mediation>.

2009, a VRI system was implemented in four general hospitals in Belgium. The results of the user assessment of the system indicated that, although nearly all health care providers, patients and intercultural mediators preferred F2FI, most of them were convinced that intercultural mediation through the internet was a valuable strategy to improve the quality of care for ethnic minority patients. The most important problem that came up in the research was the lack of familiarity with the use of videoconferencing equipment, which made the interventions lengthier and exposed the need for supplementary training on equipment use:

> VRI is more complex than face to face interpreting: important aspects are procedures to check sound and image quality at the beginning of the intervention, the moderate use of gestures, note-taking and the management of turn taking. Finally, the main issue seems to be to make health care providers familiar with the system and to make them rely on it when they encounter a linguistic or socio-cultural barrier that makes the intervention of the mediator necessary. (Verrept, 2011: 8)

This research project, which has meanwhile expanded its coverage of intercultural mediation by video link to over 160 healthcare institutions in Belgium in twenty languages (Verrept et al., 2018), was recently re-evaluated. Intercultural mediators and their managers, as well as healthcare providers, were asked to give their opinions on, among other things, the efficiency and acceptability of VI (compared with F2FI) in removing the linguistic and cultural barriers of non-Dutch-speaking patients. The data were collected by means of interviews and focus groups. The findings show that satisfaction with VI much depended on the users. Whereas healthcare providers considered VI a valuable alternative (despite their preference for F2FI), intercultural mediators considered VI an additional burden and found it more tiring, leaving them "less room to function as a mediator" (*ibid.*: 58). The re-evaluation also indicated that despite the growing number of video-link interventions, the limited willingness of managers to implement VI due to increased costs and logistical issues hinders its efficient application (*ibid.*: 59). Based on this evaluation, a number of guidelines for the organization of video remote intercultural mediation were established (Verrept & Coune, 2016). The guidelines include the obligation for intercultural mediators to use a headset, follow specific VRI training and ensure that the image and sound quality is "good" on both sides, in order to "carry out quality interpretation" (*ibid.*: 31).

Finally, the most recent study on VRI in healthcare settings, investigating authentic materials collected in hospitals in Norway, was carried out by Hansen (2020), who looked in particular into the interactional dynamics of VRI and mainly established turn-taking issues, which she linked to "asymmetry" in the participants' distribution in space. Based on the same data, Hansen and Svennevig (2021) demonstrated that, frequently, pre-beginning signals by a participant wanting to take the floor (e.g. an in-breath or opening the mouth) were not picked up by the party present in the other location, which inhibited smooth turn-taking. The authors argue that participants are often unaware of the limitations of videoconferencing technology.

OTHER SETTINGS OF DIALOGUE INTERPRETING

Davitti's (2018) study comparing VRI and F2FI in different settings of DI (parent-teacher meetings and legal interpreting) aims primarily to broaden the analytical scope to investigate DI. As the scholar argues, a fine-grained multimodal approach to DI is required to account for its interactional complexity and multilayered character. According to Davitti (*ibid.*: 7), multimodal methodology is particularly suited to investigate video-mediated DI, because "interacting via screens without sharing the same physical space adds a further layer of complexity to interactional dynamics". This is demonstrated through multimodal analyses of authentic F2FI exchanges and quasi-simulated VRI exchanges (in which the interpreters were not aware of the fact that their interpreting assignment was simulated). From these data, the implementation of "chunking" was analysed as a case in point. In DI, chunking refers to the ways in which interpreters understand on a moment-by-moment basis how and when to intervene during a multi-unit turn and how interpreters can accomplish turn allocation to the same speaker, while at the same time "ensuring a smooth communicative flow" (*ibid.*: 14). Chunking is a subtle process, established by means of embodied resources (such as gaze, gesture and head movement) and/or verbal and prosodic resources. The analyses show how in F2FI, chunking can be achieved by embodied sources only, whereas VRI poses (partial) constraints on the efficiency of the use of embodied resources only.

In the same vein, the research by Davitti and Braun (2020) in several collaborative settings of DI, such as nurse-patient interaction and customer services (taken from the Shift project mentioned earlier in this section), adopts a micro-analytical and multimodal approach to understanding interaction in VRI. On the one hand, it specifically identifies interactional issues in non-mediated communication, how they unfold in VRI and how interpreters cope with them. On the other, the analysis of the impact of possible interpreter strategies can contribute to more holistic interpreter training. The paper pays special attention to the management of the opening and closing of a communicative exchange, since in these "crucial interactional moments", rapport is established and confirmed (*ibid*.: 285). Their analyses demonstrate that in VRI, all participants make somewhat exaggerated efforts in their greetings (welcome and goodbye), for instance, by making explicit waving gestures to compensate for possible lack of rapport, which renders their behaviour somewhat "awkward". However, this "awkwardness" does not hinder the outcome of the communicative event, nor does it lead to communication breakdown. The research also observed a lack of clarity about who is to initiate and close the session. It shows that, in the data under investigation, the interpreters took up the coordinating role, which increased their visibility but also led to a certain awkwardness, as mentioned above. Altogether, the study confirms earlier studies by Braun indicating that the usual, embodied face-to-face strategies that people use in conversation may be less efficient in VRI (*ibid*.: 285).

SIGN LANGUAGE INTERPRETING (SLI)

A volume bringing together research on interpreting via video link in signed and spoken language edited by Napier et al. (2018) identifies factors that impact on the viability of VI, as well as the features that are specific to the different VI configurations (Skinner et al., 2018). In sign language interpreting, RI consists of video relay service (VRS) and video remote interpreting (VRI). In VRS, each of the participants (the deaf person, the hearing person and the interpreter) are in separate locations. They are connected via video link (the deaf person and the interpreter) and by telephone connection (the hearing person and the interpreter). By contrast, VRI in SLI is similar to VRI in spoken language interpreting, in that the deaf person and the hearing person are together at one location, whereas the interpreter is connected via video link from a separate location (*ibid.*: 17–18).

The major constraints of VI described in the studies on video relay service (VRS) are in line with the findings from research on spoken-language VI. For example, Bower (2015) identified comparable technical issues in VRS and in spoken language VI, that is, a slow internet connection causing image freezing and poor audio connection. In addition, more specific problems connecting calls due to the VRS software were observed (*ibid.*: 8). Besides technological, linguistic, interactional issues and environmental issues, Napier and Leneham (2011: 60) also describe logistical issues as an important obstacle to the success of VI in SLI, for example, a lack of briefing beforehand to inform the participants of the idiosyncrasies of the media that are used. An additional difficulty for interpreters in VRS compared with spoken-language RI is the combination of telephone and video-link use. Most of the time, the interpreter is connected to a deaf person by video link and to the hearing person by telephone (Alley, 2012). The differences encountered in sign-language RI by Napier et al. (2018) are similar to the ones described in the TI studies on spoken-language RI in dialogue settings discussed earlier in this section, such as lack of visual access to contextual cues and feelings of absence. Similarly, Warnicke and Plejert (2016: 198) demonstrate that in VRI, the sign language interpreter's positioning

> emerges dynamically in relation to contingent variables of the setting, such as the initial importance of briefing users on the service, temporary loss of sound and image, the perceived need to inform either user of extralinguistic items, or situational awareness that it is time to conclude the interaction.

Other important issues pinpointed by Napier et al. (2018: 237) are confidentiality matters, feelings of marginalization and quality of the telephone connection, as well as imbalance in experience with VRI between deaf users and the hearing party, the latter of whom are usually less familiar with this interpreting method. These various factors have consequences for the sign language interpreter's role, as demonstrated by the application of the role-space model (Llewelynn-Jones & Lee, 2014), developed to assess the visibility of the interpreter in VRS compared to F2FI.

2.3 Research issues and caveats

The literature review demonstrates that despite the different research angles and methods, many similar issues related to the use of RI were observed across interpreting settings and modes. It also shows discrepancies between subjective and objective quality assessment of RI. For example, although no objective proof was found for the psychological and physical complaints of remote conference interpreters, the interpreters actually perceived that the quality of interpreting was lower in RCI and experienced an increase of fatigue and a lack of control. By contrast, experiments in remote dialogue interpreting proved that the increased cognitive load in remote conditions led in some cases to an earlier onset of fatigue than was the case in F2FI, which resulted in an increase in miscommunication.

What all studies agree on – to a greater or lesser extent – is that the quality of TI and VI is influenced – or, at least, is perceived to be influenced – by the environment, that is, by the remote conditions. These include the technical equipment used for communication, bandwidth, connection, seating arrangement, background noise and lights. These conditions also affect interactional aspects of the interpreting process and may have an impact on the transfer of message content and the efficiency of the use of embodied resources. Moreover, in RI, compared with F2FI, the coordinating role of the interpreter has been demonstrated to be extended because of the changes in interactional dynamics. Many of the studies conclude that RI is only feasible when certain minimum standards are met and that familiarity with technology-mediated interpreting, not only by the interpreters but also by the other users of interpreting services (such as patients, clients, healthcare providers and police officers) contributes to a more efficient use of RI. Therefore, much of the research recommends additional training for an effective use of RI methods, specifically regarding interaction management.

Although the results of almost all studies indicate participant preference for F2FI, it seems logical that as the technological conditions continue to improve and users become more familiar with RI, it will have increasingly better chances for successfully achieving the specific communication goals it is used for, and of being increasingly accepted by users. Moreover, since RI is becoming more common and widespread by the day, especially since the worldwide pandemic that started in 2020, it is quite likely that professional interpreters participating in research projects today are already much more familiar with RI than the interpreters who took part in earlier research projects. Research involving more experienced remote interpreters, or younger interpreters with a higher degree of digital literacy than the generation of interpreters before them, may very well yield different results than the earlier studies.

Considering the most frequently recurring issue in the existing research, that is, the impact of the remote conditions on interpreting quality, there is one fundamental question that has only been partially answered so far: how and to what extent the remote conditions may affect the quality of RI compared with F2FI. Moreover, within the RI methods, one of the most important issues yet to be explored are the potential benefits of using an audiovisual channel compared with an audio-only channel.

Now that I have identified research issues and caveats in the field of RDI in this chapter, I will move on the discuss the methodological framework of my research (Part II), starting with the presentation of the conceptual framework underpinning the methodology of my research in Chapter 3, which investigates the concept of quality in interpreting by identifying its main components, and which explains how this concept was approached to investigate RDI in healthcare settings.

PART II

Theoretical Framework

CHAPTER 3

Investigating Quality

In this section, I discuss the conceptual framework underpinning the methodology of this research. Firstly, I address important aspects of interpreting quality (Section 3.1). Secondly, I explain why it is useful to have a multidisciplinary, holistic approach that combines insights from bilingual healthcare communication and interpreting studies to investigate the quality of remote dialogue interpreting in healthcare settings (Section 3.2).

3.1 Interpreting quality

Given that interpreting is a complex cognitive, linguistic, cultural and social process, the issue of its quality is multifaceted (Grbić, 2015). Early studies on interpreting quality focused on accuracy and fidelity in conference interpreting (Barik, 1971, 1975/2002; Gerver, 1975; Oléron & Nanpon, 1965) and in sign language interpreting (Cokely, 1992). They consisted mainly of linguistic error analyses comparing source text input and target text output, in order to identify "translation departures" (Barik, 1975/2002, in Pöchhacker 2016/2004: 137). Although source–target text correspondence has remained a central issue in the assessment of interpreting quality, leading to an overwhelming variety of models and classifications (Pöchhacker, 2016/2004: 137), the concept of interpreting quality has come to be linked to many other factors besides accuracy. For example, the cultural complexity of the interpreter's task (Kaufert & Koolage, 1984) has gained significant prominence. Also, interactional aspects of interpreter-mediated communicative events have increasingly gained interest, with, from the 1990s on, interpreting scholars shifting their attention from conference interpreting to interpreting events involving different types of dialogue interpreting (DI).

DI refers to interpreter-mediated communication involving triadic exchanges between primary participants and an interpreter (Mason, 2001). In the humanities, as language generally came to be considered a form of social interaction (Van Dijk, 1997), interpreting scholars such as Bot (2005), Davidson (2002), Mason (2001), Metzger (1999), Roy (2000), Tebble (1993) and Wadensjö (1998) turned to sociolinguistics to study DI. This methodological approach to DI is also referred to as the "dialogic discourse-based interactionist research paradigm" (Pöchhacker, 2016/2004: 75) and has become the predominant approach in investigating DI. Within this paradigm, the coordination of the communication, or interaction management, is an important factor in the assessment of interpreting quality.

Figure 2 represents the most important elements specifically related to DI that are relevant to the assessment of remote healthcare interpreting, particularly from a discourse-analytical perspective. The model proposed here is by no means comprehensive, but aims to integrate the various aspects of interpreting quality in DI that fall within the scope of this research.

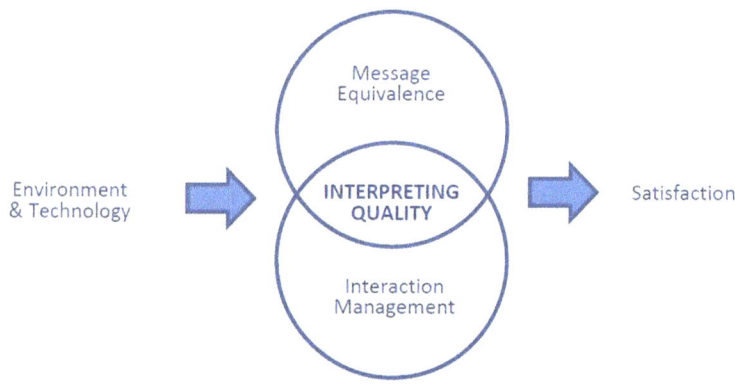

Figure 2. Quality of remote dialogue interpreting.

In the model shown in Figure 2, interpreting quality is viewed as a combination of two major components, that is, the interpreter's performance in terms of message equivalence and the participants' interaction management. This model is based on Wadensjö's (1998: 105) assumption of the two central tasks of the interpreter, that is, the translation and the coordination of the primary participants' utterances. As Wadensjö (*ibid.*: 105) argues, in DI, "the translating and coordinating aspects are *simultaneously present*, and the one does not exclude the other, as a matter of fact, these aspects condition each other".

Message equivalence (translation) and interaction management (coordination) are in turn influenced by the environmental and technological conditions in which interpreter-mediated communication takes place. Lastly, the quality of interpreter-mediated communication is expressed in the satisfaction of the participants in the communication. Given that satisfaction with the communication is key to establishing rapport between the participants, examining users' perceptions is extremely useful in assessing the effectiveness of the communication. In healthcare settings specifically, satisfaction and trust in the doctor–patient relationship and in clinical outcomes rely primarily on effective communication (Anazawa et al., 2012).

In the following sections, we will elaborate on the concepts of message equivalence and interaction management and explain how these two components, vital in assessing the quality of interpreter-mediated healthcare communication, are interrelated.

3.1.1 *Message equivalence*

As mentioned in this section's introduction, in interpreting studies, the correspondence between the source text and its rendition in the target language, to which we will refer as "message equivalence", remains a central issue in the assessment of the interpreting performance (Pöchhacker, 2016/2004). Ever since Herbert's (1952) description of the interpreter's task as "fully and faithfully" conveying a speaker's message, researchers have reflected on how exactly to define message equivalence. One of its most prominent characteristics seems to be accuracy. As Tiselius and

Englund Dimitrova (2016) argue, the requirement of accuracy is mentioned in many codes of conduct, although there is little agreement on what the term actually comprises. Accuracy measurement often uses taxonomies to describe and quantify different components, such as omission, addition, substitution and fluency. Over time, many different taxonomies have been developed to measure message equivalence at several levels, far beyond the transfer of propositional content. When conveying messages from one participant to the other, interpreters must produce renditions that reflect the source message's content at the levels of information and pragmatics (propositional content and intentional effect), as well as at the level of form and the speaker level (linguistic structure and style) (Van der Kleij, 2015). The need to consider style as an inherent aspect of message equivalence has been claimed by several researchers, such as Angelelli (2004), Gile (1992) and Hatim and Mason (1990). Style is expressed in both nonverbal and verbal acts, as well as in linguistic and paralinguistic cues. It includes affective elements and specific source message characteristics such as register, which give meaning to the message (Wadensjö, 1998).

Besides transferring message content and style, achieving message equivalence also includes managing the emotive character of the interlocutors' speech, by making cues that convey affect accessible to the interlocutors (Cirillo, 2010). The same applies to empathic cues. Empathy refers to the ability to understand another person's situation, perspectives and feelings, including the meanings attached to these, as well as the ability to communicate that understanding and act on that understanding in a helpful way (Mercer & Reynolds, 2002; Morse et al., 1992). This is considered a basic element of any therapeutic relationship (Reynolds et al., 1999). Hale (2007) adds to this topic by exploring the ethical dimension of message equivalence. She states that achieving accuracy is especially important in healthcare settings, since in this context, health outcomes are at stake.

In terms of assessing message equivalence, many researchers have pointed out that this can only be achieved by taking into account contextual factors. Wadensjö (1998) uses the concept of "closeness" as an indication of source–target text correspondence at a linguistic and cultural and interactional level. Her research, based on transcriptions of authentic interpreting sessions in community settings, distinguishes between two types of interpreter contributions: renditions and non-renditions.

Renditions represent original utterances and can, in the scholar's taxonomy, be close (equivalent to the original utterance at the level of content, style and interaction), expanded (containing more content than the original utterance), reduced (containing less content than the original utterance), substituting (a combination of expanded and reduced renditions) or summarizing (an interlocutor's original utterance is summarized rather than rendered as a whole). Additionally, there can be a lack of rendition, which Wadensjö refers to as a "zero rendition". Non-renditions are utterances by the interpreter that are not renditions of the primary participants' original utterances and usually have a coordinating function. Wadensjö (*ibid.*) concludes that interpreters do not necessarily produce perfectly matching renditions at a word-by-word or sentence level, but rather convey messages that meet the interlocutors' communicative goals within the larger interactional context. Napier (2004) builds on this concept by demonstrating that certain types of omission are a result of strategic decision-making and do not necessarily imply a decrease in accuracy. In the same vein, Major and Napier (2012: 211) point out that specifically in healthcare settings

> judgments of accuracy should be made based on wider contextual evidence. Studies based on authentic spoken and signed language interpreting data have provided evidence that strategic decisionmaking, based on contextual factors, is a key component in healthcare interpreting.

In their study on sign language interpreting between English and Australian Sign Language, Major and Napier (*ibid.: 209*) apply Wadensjö's taxonomy, based on a corpus of simulated doctor–patient interaction. Its results provide further evidence that error-based taxonomies of accuracy are insufficient to explain strategic decision-making by interpreters and that accuracy in healthcare settings must be assessed within the interactional context of the interpreter-mediated event.

3.1.2 Interaction management

The importance that interpreting scholars attach to context in assessing message equivalence is in line with the aforementioned discourse-based interactionist approach that predominates in DI research and which is also adopted in the current work. In this approach, the ways in which the interaction management unfolds in DI events is a main point of interest. To study interaction management, different frameworks within discourse analysis are applied. As Hale (2007: 204–205) remarks, combinations of discourse-analytical frameworks are often applied in DI studies. This has led to a rather eclectic application of this theory, ranging from conversation analysis (CA) and interactional sociolinguistics to micro-linguistic and critical discourse analysis.

Discourse-based interactional approaches generally follow the basic CA principles claiming that participants organize their speech in a systematic way (Sacks et al., 1974) and that that utterances and actions can only be understood within the context in which they occur (Heath, 2004/1986). According to CA principles, conversations are sequentially organized, that is, interlocutors coordinate their interaction by building on previous utterances. This is most clearly demonstrated by the CA notion of "adjacency pairs" (Schegloff, 1972). Adjacency pairs are sequences that consist of two parts, the latter of which depends on the former one. In other words, the production of the first part of an adjacency pair creates the expectation that the second part will occur, for example, in the case of a question-/answer sequence, or mutual greetings. Through systematic examinations of naturally occurring conversation, Sacks et al. (1974) also determined that there are general rules underlying the coordination of conversation. Among these principles are, for example, the observation that participants generally speak one at the time, that overlapping speech is common but brief, and that turn transitions may be accompanied by pauses in the form of gaps and overlaps (*ibid.*).

The concept of turn-taking is central to the study of interaction management. Turn-taking is considered a basic characteristic of dialogue, which is central to the discourse process and demonstrates its interactional character (*ibid.*: 728). Studies on this concept look at how participants jointly determine who will speak and who will listen, and how transitions in the participation framework are achieved (Goffman, 1981; Gumperz, 1982; Sacks et al., 1974; Schiffrin, 1994). The participants' collaborative work in constructing turns systematically modifies the structure of each sentence "by adding to it, deleting from it, and changing its meaning" (Goodwin,

1979: 112). In this way, speakers' actions are both context-shaped and context-renewing (Heritage & Maynard, 2006: 10–11).

The discourse-based approach was adopted by interpreting scholars investigating interpreter-mediated events involving people from different communities that do not share the same language and culture (Hale, 2007). For this activity, an almost infinite number of terms can be found in the literature, ranging from community interpreting to public service interpreting, liaison interpreting, bilateral interpreting, triad interpreting and dialogue interpreting (Hsieh, 2016; Tipton & Furmanek, 2016), to name but a few. The most common names seem to be "community interpreting" and "public service interpreting", which are used interchangeably in ISO 18841 ("General requirements and recommendations for interpreting services", 2018) and defined as "interpreting that enables people to access services available to society as a whole, and which they would otherwise be unable to access owing to a language barrier" (*ibid.*: 3). More specifically, in ISO 13611 ("Guidelines for community interpreting", 2014), community interpreting is described as "a profession, not as an informal practice such as interpreting performed by friends, family members, children" (*ibid.*: n.p.).

In this work, we will henceforth use the term "dialogue interpreting" (DI), coined by Mason (1999), to refer to interpreter-mediated communication involving triadic exchanges between primary participants and an interpreter. This term highlights the interactive and dynamic nature of this type of event (Hsieh, 2016), as opposed to the mostly unidirectional character of other types of interpreting, such as conference interpreting (Davitti, 2018).

In line with the discourse-based perspective, interpreter scholars have demonstrated – by means of elaborate descriptions of turn-taking in interpreter-mediated communication, also called triadic communication – that the interpreter is an extra link in the interactional turn-taking chain. As we have seen, managing interaction is considered an essential aspect of the interpreter's task. The interpreter thus plays a pivotal role, both as the facilitator of dialogue between participants from separate linguistic and cultural communities, and as a conversation manager. Interpreters, just like the primary participants, shift between different roles, expressed through their acts of translating, requesting and providing clarifications, engaging in nonverbal behaviour, et cetera. Through these actions, the interpreter contributes, both verbally and nonverbally, to the primary participants' interaction and to the negotiation of meaning (Bot, 2005; Krystallidou, 2014, 2016; Mason, 2001; Roy, 2000; Wadensjö, 1998).

The coordination of the interaction can be implicit or explicit (Wadensjö, 1998). Whereas implicit coordination refers to regular turn-taking, that is, when the interpreter has his or her turn immediately after one of the primary participants' turns (Roy, 2000), explicit coordination takes place when regular turn-taking is temporarily abandoned, for example, when the interpreter initiates a turn by requesting clarification. This is what Wadensjö (1998) calls an "explicit non-rendition". Baraldi and Gavioli (2014) further refined Wadensjö's notions of coordination by introducing the terms "basic" and "reflexive" coordination to describe the interaction management in interpreter-mediated communication. According to them, these terms are needed to demonstrate that interaction management and message equivalence are very closely connected and that coordination cannot be separated from content. Baraldi and Gavioli (*ibid.*: 336) explain that source–target text correspondence is achieved through accuracy in the transfer of content and by means of coordinating activities:

> For renditions to be 'close' […], interpreting mediators need to achieve 'accurate' coordination work [as] […] closeness in meaning and function in single utterances does not necessarily coincide with closeness in their function in the interaction.

Baraldi and Gavioli (2012) point out that implicit and explicit coordination may overlap, because explicit non-renditions often pertain to the interpreter's ability to deliver an accurate rendition. Therefore, the interruption is relevant to the interpreting task (Mason & Rock, 2019). Moreover, as Baraldi and Gavioli (2012) argue, by choosing a specific format in which to render an utterance, interpreters also coordinate the interaction, without explicitly altering the process of regular turn-taking. This is what they refer to as reflexive coordination, whereas basic coordination is considered a form of implicit coordination (i.e. regular turn-taking) that does not involve explicit coordinating intentions.

How interpreters cope with interaction management depends not only on their own skills, but also on the behaviour, expectations and goals of the primary participants. As Wadensjö (1998) argues, together, the primary participants and interpreter form an interactional chain, which she calls a "communicative radius" or "pas de trois", in which each link is responsible for the interaction. In the same vein, Roy (2000: 68) introduces the concept of "interactional harmony": "the participants, the discourse, and the moment combine [...] to create interactional harmony whereby a turn happens successfully and comfortably".

This "interactional harmony" can take place because of the participants' ability to indicate and recognize so-called "transition relevance places", or TRP's (Sacks et al., 1974). These are potential possibilities for turn transition. This ability is essential in achieving smooth turn-taking (Bot, 2005). As Sacks et al. (1974) explain, speakers design their turns in a way that other participants can follow their intentions. They do so, for example, by inserting pauses, by their lexical choices, voice intonation or by shifting their gaze. As research in interpreting studies has amply demonstrated (Bot, 2005; Roy, 2000), interpreters are actively involved in achieving smooth turn transitions by monitoring these verbal and nonverbal turn-transition signals. The combined verbal and nonverbal resources used for the coordination of interaction are examples of the multimodal character of communication.

Over the years, the seminal work by Sacks et al. (1974) that constitutes the basis of the discourse-based interactional approach has been further complemented and refined, especially by means of ever-more fine-grained accounts of the multimodal character of dialogue. Studies on interaction management in monolingual conversation such as Bavelas et al. (2002), Heath (2004/1986), Kendon (1967), Kress and Van Leeuwen (2001), Mondada (2016) and Rossano et al. (2009) have increasingly focused on the role of participants' nonverbal behaviour in conversation, for example, to steer the interaction. Moreover, the introduction of innovative research methods such as mobile eye-tracking (Vranjes, 2018; Vranjes et al., 2019) has led to more fine-grained accounts of the role of gaze, gesture, body posture, proxemics, the handling of artefacts and spatial arrangement in interaction (Davitti & Pasquandrea, 2017), taking into account the multimodal character of conversation.

Multimodality is a broad theoretical concept that comprises several methodological frameworks. In general, multimodal theories consider that interaction between participants occurs through a combination of different communicative resources or "communication modes" (Norris, 2004, 2009), or, in the words of Stivers and Sidnell (2005: 2): "Participants [in interaction] encounter a steady stream of meaningful facial expressions, gestures, body postures, head movements, words, grammatical constructions, and prosodic contours."

An important principle in multimodal theory is that no semiotic resources are prioritized over others. Instead, they are considered intertwined layers in the complex interactional process between participants (Pasquandrea, 2011: 457), who use a multitude of semiotic resources to convey meaning and monitor comprehension (Kress & Van Leeuwen, 2001; Mondada, 2016). Speakers can, for example, use gesture to emphasize their intentions. At the same time, they may gaze at listeners to assess the reception of their message as expressed by these through posture, gesture, facial expression, etc. (Bavelas et al., 2002). In particular, gaze direction and mutual gaze between participants, which is also referred to as "gaze window" (*ibid.*), can play an important role in the coordination of the interaction, as well as in the expression of involvement in the communication (Kendon, 1967; Rossano et al., 2009).

Multimodal approaches were introduced in interpreting studies by scholars such as Davitti (2013), Davitti and Pasquandrea (2017), Krystallidou (2014), Mason (2012), Monteoliva-García (2020), Pasquandrea (2011) and Vranjes (2018). Their studies have provided highly detailed analyses of interaction management in DI and generated useful insights in the role of gaze, gesture, body posture, proxemics, artefact handling and spatial arrangement in DI interactions (Davitti & Pasquandrea, 2017).

By describing interaction management from a discourse-based, multimodal approach, interpreting scholars have not only provided insight into the ways in which understanding in mediated discourse is achieved interactionally, but also how it is conditioned by the sociocultural settings in which DI takes place (Wadensjö, 1998), that is, the discourse context.

From a discourse-based approach, the context in which the communication takes place must be borne in mind when evaluating the quality of interpreter-mediated communication. The discourse context is the larger, overall institutional or social context in which the interpreter-mediated communication is embedded (Angelelli, 2004). Since my research focuses on healthcare settings, this section is limited to this particular type of discourse context.

Just like other institutional communicative events, medical consultations are a specific "genre" (Eggins, 1994), meaning that this type of event has a specific purpose and consists of schematic procedures that both determine and constrain choices in terms of content, lexis, syntax and style (Swales, 1990). One of the most obvious characteristics of doctor–patient interaction is the structure of the medical consultation, which consists of different phases, or genre steps (Tebble, 2014), each of which involves its own specific communication dynamics (Byrne & Long, 1984/1976; Heath, 1992, 1986/2004; Heritage & Maynard, 2006). The structure of doctor–patient consultations can be divided into five genre steps: (1) opening phase, (2) problem presentation, (3) verbal and/or physical examination, (4) diagnosis, treatment and check-ups, and (5) closing (Byrne & Long, 1984/1976; Heritage & Maynard, 2006).

As Tebble (2014: 418) points out, understanding the "social purpose and discourse structure of specific professional speech events" can teach interpreting students how to interpret the communicative goals, content and discourse manners of both service providers and clients. Therefore, knowledge of the specific dynamics implicit to the discourse environment is essential for interpreters and interpreting students (Baraldi & Gavioli, 2012, 2014; Tebble, 1993, 1999, 2012, 2014).

3.2 Remote healthcare interpreting: A holistic approach

As Hsieh (2016: 9) puts forward, interpreter-mediated healthcare encounters represent an interdisciplinary research field situated at "the intersection of languages, cultures, and medicine, all of which entail distinct values and norms". When assessing the quality or "successfulness" of interpreter-mediated healthcare communication (Hsieh, 2017; Meeuwesen, 2010), we must attempt to respect its multifaceted character as much as possible. In order to open the investigation of the quality of (remote) healthcare interpreting to a wide range of linguistic and interactional considerations, this study combines discourse-based and multimodal approaches in interpreting studies (Angelelli, 2004; Baraldi & Gavioli, 2012, 2014; Davitti, 2012, 2013, 2018; Davitti & Pasquandrea, 2017; Krystallidou, 2014, Tebble, 1999; Valero-Garcés, 2005) with insights from bilingual healthcare communication (Harmsen et al., 2005; Hsieh, 2007, 2017; Hsieh & Hong, 2010; Hsieh & Kramer, 2021; Meeuwesen et al., 2010; Schouten et al., 2020). Notions of research on social interaction, as described in Section 3.2 (Heath, 2004/1986, 1992; Heritage & Maynard, 2006; Mondada, 2007, 2011, 2016; Sacks et al., 1974), are also taken into consideration. Throughout this work, the terms "quality" and "success" of the communication are used interchangeably.

In interpreting studies, healthcare interpreting is one of the most prevalent fields of professional practice and research within the overarching category of DI (Hale, 2007; Pöchhacker & Schlesinger, 2005). It is a very broad label, covering diverse types of interpreter-mediated interactions involving medical professionals ranging from doctors, physiotherapists, nurses and midwives, to speech pathologists, mental healthcare providers and so forth (Ng & Crezee, 2020; Tipton & Furmanek, 2016). A general definition that applies to all these types of interpreting is provided by Angelelli (2014: 574), who describes healthcare interpreting as an interaction occurring between three parties, that is, "a speaker of a non-societal language (for example a patient seeking healthcare)", "a speaker of the societal language (generally the service provider)" and an interpreter, "who mediates between the two parties in a simultaneous or consecutive mode, either face-to-face or remotely".

As we saw in Section 3.1.2 (Interaction management), researchers adhering to a discourse-based approach to DI put forward that both the primary parties and the interpreter jointly contribute to the process and outcome of the communication. This is particularly the case in healthcare interpreting (Angelelli, 2007). From the same perspective, Pittarello (2012) argues that the ways in which participants organize their interaction in terms of turn-taking and communication exchanges contributes to the success or failure of the interaction. In other words:

> The outcome of interpreter-mediated interaction is the result of a subtle combination and balancing out of strategies adopted and choices made by the interpreter and by the participants in a constant process of interactional negotiation. (Davitti, 2012: 24)

Therefore, in evaluating the successfulness of intercultural communication management in healthcare settings, the interactional behaviour of all participants must be taken into account. The view that interpreter-mediated communication is interactionally achieved is confirmed by research from the perspective of bilingual healthcare communication. In this discipline, researchers often relate to the quality of communication in terms of the successfulness of the communication (Hsieh, 2017; Meeuwesen, 2010). Hsieh (2017) argues that the interpersonal dynamics between the healthcare provider, the patient and the interpreter may shape the process and content of interpreter-mediated medical encounters. This is confirmed by other researchers in bilingual healthcare communication, such as Gerwing and Li (2019: 174), who claim that conversations are collaborative and coordinated activities in which the actions of the participants are mutually influential.

Regardless of which research perspective is adopted and of whether we talk about the quality' or success of interpreter-mediated communication, we can assume that the purpose of healthcare communication that is mediated by professional interpreters is to achieve effective communication in terms of mutual understanding between the patient and the healthcare provider. From the perspective of healthcare communication studies, three aspects that can affect the successfulness of the interpreter-mediated interventions are: (1) miscommunication (i.e. misunderstanding and other communication problems), (2) changes in translation and (3) side-talk activities (Meeuwesen et al., 2010: 202). These indicators correspond to the two important dimensions of interpreting quality as considered from the perspective of interpreting studies, as discussed earlier in this section (Baraldi & Gavioli, 2012, 2014; Hatim & Mason, 1990; Metzger, 1999; Roy, 2000; Wadensjo, 1998), that is, message equivalence and interaction management (Figure 2). These two aspects also represent the dual service the interpreter must give, firstly, providing an accurate and adequate equivalent of a source text and, secondly, ensuring successful interaction (Pöchhacker, 2001).

In this research, we combine the perspectives outlined above. To assess the quality of interpreter-mediated interaction, we investigate the achievement of mutual understanding, firstly by examining miscommunication by looking into issues at the levels of message equivalence and interaction.

Secondly, since communication takes place within a specific interactional context that affects the communication, we look specifically into the ways in which the interaction is managed. For this purpose, besides the translational activities, we examine actions other than translating, that is, repair of miscommunication and communication aimed to optimize reaching a mutual understanding. Thirdly, factors independent of the participants, such as contextual issues (e.g. noise from the environment, seating arrangement) and the technological conditions in which the interpreter-mediated communication takes place (e.g. sound and image quality, position within camera view) are studied, since these may also directly or indirectly influence the successfulness of the communication. The ways in which these concepts related to quality are operationalized in the research design are explained in the next chapter (Chapter 4), which outlines this research's methodology.

CHAPTER 4

Methodology

This chapter presents the methodology that was used for investigating remote healthcare interpreting from a holistic perspective. It starts with a presentation of the general outline of the research and the questions that are central to the research (Section 4.1). After that, I explain how the data were collected (Section 4.2), how they were prepared for the analysis by means of the design of annotation categories (Section 4.3), and, finally, how the data were analysed (Section 4.4).

4.1 General outline and research questions

As we have seen in the literature review in Chapter 2, the diversity in the research design and perspectives in medical studies and interpreting studies on RI in healthcare settings leaves us with many contradictory results and questions yet to be answered. As far as the actual situation in healthcare interpreting is concerned, there is a growing practice of – and demand for – integrating remote interpreting (RI) methods next to face-to-face (consecutive) interpreting (F2FI). In this context, we summarize four of the most important issues requiring further research. First, a comparative analysis is needed of possible differences in quality between the F2FI method and the different RI methods telephone interpreting (TI) and video interpreting (VI). Secondly, we need to gain clearer insight into the remote conditions' impact on the success of interpreter-mediated communication. Thirdly, differences in interactional dynamics between the F2FI and RI methods and the relationship between issues occurring at different levels (message equivalence, interaction and technology) are in need of further exploration. A fourth issue that needs to be examined within the RI methods (TI and VI) is the possible added value of the audiovisual channel compared with the audio-only channel.

To address these issues, I developed a research design consisting of simulations of doctor–patient visits mediated by three interpreters, each performing her task in the consecutive mode using three different interpreting methods: (1) face-to-face interpreting (F2FI), (2) telephone interpreting (TI) and (3) video interpreting (VI). Every interpreter experienced all three interpreting methods. The data collected from the simulations (nine altogether) were systematically annotated, analysed and compared. After each simulation, all three participants were interviewed to collect their perceptions on (1) the quality of the interpreting, (2) the quality of the communication, (3) the quality of the healthcare provided, (4) their satisfaction with the technological conditions and the seating arrangement and (5) their preferred interpreting method. Two weeks after the simulations, the three interpreters were interviewed again and asked to comment on specific issues that were observed in a first, basic analysis of the video data. The results from the video data analysis were cross-referenced with the results of the analyses from the participants' perceptions. Before providing details on the research design and data analysis, first the conceptual approach underpinning this work will be explained.

To evaluate the quality of the different interpreting methods in healthcare communication, we must attempt to respect its multifaceted character as much as possible. In line with the focus of this research, the following five research questions were formulated:

1. Are there differences in quality in interpreter-mediated doctor–patient communication between the three interpreting methods under investigation (F2FI, TI, VI), as expressed by the number and nature of issues at the level of message equivalence and/or at the level of interaction?
2. Are there differences in interaction management in interpreter-mediated doctor–patient communication between the three

interpreting methods F2FI, TI and VI, as expressed by the number and nature of repair and optimization strategies?
3. Is there a relationship between message equivalence issues and interactional issues?
4. Can possible differences in quality between the RI methods (TI, VI) and the F2FI method be attributed to environmental and/or technological factors?
5. Within the RI methods (TI, VI), are there benefits to the quality of the communication when using an audiovisual channel (VI) in comparison with an audio-only channel (TI)?

To answer these questions, we compared interpreter-mediated interaction across the three interpreting methods. This comparative method, which is frequently used in research on remote interpreting (RI) in both medical studies (Hornberger et al., 1996; Nápoles et al., 2010; Price Leemann et al., 2012; Saint-Louis et al., 2003) and interpreting studies (Balogh & Hertog, 2012; Wang & Fang, 2019), is a useful approach for investigating the impact of the remote conditions on the communication, while at the same time overcoming the idiosyncrasies of the individual interpreters and primary participants. Despite the artificial nature of simulations, this option was chosen, because simulations allow for systematic comparison of different interpreting methods used by different interpreters. Moreover, in this way, potential difficulties associated with obtaining ethics approval for using authentic data were avoided. Following previous research on VI in legal settings (Balogh & Hertog, 2012), various settings of video-mediated DI (Davitti, 2018) and sign language interpreting (SLI) (Major & Napier, 2012), I opted for non-scripted or semi-scripted simulations, which have proven to be a successful means of comparing various interpreting methods. As Davitti (2018: 18) points out, the use of simulations or partial simulations involving professionals (such as police officers or doctors) and interpreters is a "fairly common practice" in the study of DI, mostly because of the "sensitivity and confidentiality" of authentic data. Lastly, Braun (2013: 205) draws attention to the fact that simulations allow for a "controlled environment" in which specific problems can be isolated.

4.2 Data collection

The data set consisted of nine simulations, twenty-seven post-simulation interviews and three retrospective interviews. Three different experienced and qualified dialogue interpreters participated in the simulations based on three non-scripted scenarios. Each interpreter performed in three simulations, each using three different interpreting methods (F2FI, TI, VI), together with a professional, practising gynaecologist and a simulated patient. In Sections 4.2.1–4.2.6, I discuss the details of the data collection, starting with a description of the time and place of the simulations, the participants, the scenarios and order of the simulations, the equipment that was used for the recordings, and the transcription and translation procedures.

4.2.1 Time and place

The simulations and the interviews took place at two offices at two campuses of the University of Antwerp, Belgium.[1] Prior to the simulations, all participants signed informed consent forms. Series 1 was implemented in October 2016, Series 2 and 3 in April 2017. Series 1 was originally planned as a pilot study, with the idea of using the collected data if the implementation was successful. Since this was the case, apart from some minor inconveniences (described in Sections 4.2.3 and 4.2.5), it was decided to use the data collected in Series 1 and implement Series 2 and 3 under similar conditions. However, based on the implementation of Series 1, the duration of the subsequent simulations was reduced. This will be explained in section discussing the scenarios and order of the simulations.

---

1 To provide similar experimental conditions, the location was originally supposed to be limited to one campus. However, this turned out to be impossible, since in between Series 1 and 2, the campus was relocated as a result of the Department of Translation and Interpreting's integration into the campus of the Faculty of Arts of the University of Antwerp.

Methodology

4.2.2 *Participants*

To guarantee the recruitment of only highly qualified and experienced interpreters who were active in the field, the selection of the three interpreters was based on the following five criteria:

1. Female[2] interpreter currently working as a community/healthcare interpreter;
2. Minimum of five years' experience in healthcare interpreting;
3. Holder of a master's degree in languages or interpreting;
4. Professional with specific interpreting training;
5. Member of a professional interpreting organization.

All three interpreters were found through the professional organizations of which they were members. As far as their normal working conditions were concerned, the three interpreters claimed to work mostly in F2FI and to accept TI assignments on a regular basis. Interpreter 1 also occasionally practised business interpreting via videoconferencing, whereas Interpreters 2 and 3 had never interpreted through videoconferencing before, but were familiar with videoconferencing for personal purposes.

The role of gynaecologist was performed by a qualified gynaecologist employed in a hospital in the Netherlands, who had approximately ten years of professional experience. The gynaecologist had previously worked with interpreters, although not on a regular basis. She had mostly worked with either informal interpreters or professional telephone interpreters and was familiar with videoconferencing for personal purposes.

The simulated patients were professional actors with experience as simulated patients during exams in medical studies. Contrary to what was originally planned, the simulated patient was a different person in Series 1 and in Series 2 and 3, since the first actor cancelled shortly before

---

2   To avoid possible interference of gender variety in comparing the performances of the interpreters, we chose to recruit only female interpreters. Moreover, since the subject matter of the consultations concerned gynaecology, in this way we avoided possible awkwardness of a male interpreter mediating the communication on female physiology between a female patient and a female doctor.

the planned date of the simulations of Series 2 and 3. However, intensive briefing sessions took place between the new actor and the actor in Series 1. The new actor also studied the videos of Series 1 closely, to be able to perform in more or less the same way as the first actor had. Both actors were also familiar with videoconferencing.

The language combination that was used in the simulations was French–Dutch. The doctor was a native speaker of Dutch with non-specialized language proficiency in French. The simulated patient was a native speaker of French with limited knowledge of Dutch.

4.2.3 Scenarios and simulation order

To increase authenticity, the simulations were designed around three common themes in real-life gynaecology practice. This was made possible with the help of a second professional gynaecologist. The three main themes were (1) weak pelvic floor, (2) heavy menstrual bleeding and (3) pregnancy/infertility. For each theme, three scenarios (A/B/C) were created (Table 1). Each of these scenarios contained slightly different descriptions of the patient's personal circumstances. Opting for three scenarios for each theme made it possible to avoid the participants having too much familiarity with any specific scenario. To leave room for spontaneous interaction between the participants, the scripts contained only the minimally required information. As is illustrated in Table 1, in each of the series, the order in which the scenarios were played was deliberately changed to avoid starting and finishing with the same interpreting method, which might have distorted the data regarding the precise influence of the remote conditions. This choice was based on the outcomes of previous research (Braun, 2004), which demonstrated that fatigue and cognitive overload increase as the interpreting session progresses in duration. In the qualitative analyses, the order of the simulations was kept in mind.

Table 1. Distribution of the scenarios across the series and conditions

	Theme 1: Weak pelvic floor	Theme 2: Heavy menstrual bleeding	Theme 3: Pregnancy/ infertility
Series 1 (Interpreter 1)	F2FI-1 scenario 1A	VI-1 scenario 2B	TI-1 scenario 3C
Series 2 (Interpreter 2)	TI-2 scenario 1B	F2FI-2 scenario 2C	VI-2 scenario 3A
Series 3 (Interpreter 3)	VI-3 scenario 1C	TI-3 scenario 2A	F2FI-3 scenario 3B

Note. F2FI = face-to-face interpreting, TI = telephone interpreting, VI = video interpreting

Table 1 shows, for example, that Series 1 (involving Interpreter 1) started with the F2FI method. For this simulation, scenario 1A ("weak pelvic floor") was used. The second simulation by Interpreter 1 was implemented in VI, using scenario 2B ("heavy menstrual bleeding"). Lastly, the third simulation by Interpreter 1 was in TI, based on Scenario 3C ("pregnancy/infertility").

The doctor and the patient each received a basic scenario (Table 2a), as well as an individual oral briefing on their roles. The doctor was given instructions to proceed as she would in her daily practice, whereas the simulated patient was given a list of complaints (Table 2b) that she had to present. The interpreters were informed only about the themes of the simulations.

Table 2a. Basic scenario 1A, F2FI-1

Ms. Fleuri, a 40-year-old French-speaking mother of three children, is referred to the gynaecologist by her general practitioner with complaints that indicate a weak pelvic floor. She has recently moved to the Netherlands for her work but does not yet speak the language. The hospital has called in an interpreter. The patient does not take any special medication.
The doctor questions the patient, explains what could be the cause of the complaints and refers her to the "Bekkenbodemcentrum", a centre specialized in pelvic floor problems. The doctor also explains what the Centre for pelvic floor problems does and provides information on incontinence products. She has also prepared a list of internet links in French about incontinence for the patient.

Table 2b. List of complaints scenario 1A, F2FI-1

Urine leakage, especially during exercise, sneezing and coughing;
Abdominal pain, fatigue and groin, leg or lower back pain;
Difficulties urinating;
Inability to empty the bladder;
Multiple bladder infections;
Frequent or short urination (overactive bladder);
Inability to hold stools;
Reduced sensitivity during sexual intercourse.

4.2.4 Duration

The duration of the simulations was initially set at approximately 20 minutes, which is the usual length of a consultation of this type in the hospital in the Netherlands in which the participating doctor worked. However, after implementing the simulations in Series 1, this consultation length turned out to be quite exhausting for the participants. Since Series 2 and 3 would have been even more tiring for the doctor and the patient, as they were implemented on the same day, the doctor received new instructions to reduce the duration to approximately 15 minutes for Series 2 and 3 (while of course following the usual structure of the consultation). As will be explained in Section 4.4.1, for the analysis of the simulations, these were divided into three parts: opening, body and closing. Tables 3–6 show the duration of the bodies, the opening and closing phases in the three series and the average full-turn duration of the bodies.

Table 3. Duration body (in minutes:seconds)

	Interpreting method		
	F2FI	TI	VI
Series 1	23:59	29:32	25:01
Series 2	20:50	16:40	25:27
Series 3	15:21	15:37	14:54

Methodology

Table 3 shows considerable variation between Series 1, 2 and 3 in the duration of the body of each simulation. This was not only the result of the decision to shorten the duration after Series 1, but also the use of non-scripted scenarios that allowed for a more natural interaction. Another explanation for the differences in the total duration of the simulations between the series was related to interpreting style. Each of the three different interpreters performing in the simulations had her own particular style of interpreting. For example, Interpreter 3 had an extremely fast way of interpreting, leaving little or no gap between the primary participants' turns and her renditions, which contributed to the shorter duration of the consultations in Series 3.

Table 4. Duration opening (in minutes:seconds)

	Interpreting method		
	F2FI	TI	VI
Series 1	01:10	02:10	01:46
Series 2	00:08	01:20	00:23
Series 3	00:37	00:43	00:40

Table 4 shows that in Series 3, there were very few differences between the interpreting methods in terms of opening duration, whereas in Series 1 and 2, the differences between the interpreting methods were considerable. Series 1 and 2 also show similarities in opening duration, with the longest openings occurring in TI and the shortest in F2FI.

Table 5. Duration closing (in minutes:seconds)

	Interpreting method		
	F2FI	TI	VI
Series 1	00:43	01:00	00:14
Series 2	01:05	00:19	00:12
Series 3	00:14	00:12	00:13

In terms of closings (Table 5), there were again hardly any differences in duration between the interpreting methods in Series 3, whereas in Series 1, the longest closing duration occurred in TI, and in Series 2, in was in F2FI.

In order to compare turn-taking patterns and interactional dynamics across the interpreting methods and interpreters, the average length of full turns in the consultations was examined. In the calculation of the average turn duration (Table 6), only floor-taking full turns were taken into account, whereas reactive tokens were not considered separate turns in the calculation. This allowed for a clearer comparison of the average turn length between the simulations, since the use of reactive tokens, which were often expressed during the interpreters' turns, varied greatly between the simulations.

Table 6. Overview of average full-turn length in body (in seconds and milliseconds)

	Interpreting method		
	F2FI	TI	VI
Series 1	23 sec 59	15 sec 82	14 sec 32
Series 2	14 sec 21	9 sec 65	16 sec 67
Series 3	9 sec 33	15 sec 65	08 sec 31

Table 6 shows no clear pattern in the average full-turn duration across the different series and interpreting methods. In Series 1, the longest average turn duration occurred in F2FI, whereas in Series 2, it was in VI and in Series 3, the longest turns were in TI. Since the doctor and patient were more-or-less constant variables, because their roles were performed by the same people or in a similar style throughout all of the simulations, the difference in average turn length seemed to depend more on the personal style of the interpreter. For example, Interpreters 1 and 2 allowed the participants to take long turns and waited for the participants to finish their turns. By contrast, Interpreter 3 (except in TI) often started her renditions before the participants had finished, forcing them to take shorter turns.

Methodology

4.2.5 Equipment and recordings

The interpreting room was equipped with a telephone and a laptop with a webcam, whereas in the doctor's room there was a telephone with speaker function, as well as a tablet, which was placed on a moveable display. The use of a speakerphone was preferred over the telephone being handed back and forth between doctor and patient, because the latter practice appeared more problematic in studies reported on by, for example, Ko (2006). For the telephone connection, a local landline was used. For the VI sessions, although it had been arranged and tested well in advance, the use of a dedicated platform with the videoconferencing software Vidyo, provided by a professional interpreting agency, had to be abandoned during the implementation of Series 1 because of connectivity problems. As a result, Skype video calling was used, which consequently was repeated for the remaining six simulations in Series 2 and 3 to maintain consistent experimental conditions. At the interpreter's location, a Sony Vaio laptop, model SV152C29M was used, whereas in the doctor's room, an iPad tablet was used, installed on a moveable display. The interpreters were given the choice whether or not to use a headset, which they all declined, citing reasons such as feeling awkward or unnatural while wearing headsets.

All simulations and interviews were recorded. The interviews and in-depth telephone interviews conducted with the interpreters two weeks after the simulation were audio-recorded, whereas the simulations themselves were video-recorded on three different cameras. The participants were captured from three different angles to allow for detailed and multimodal analyses. During F2FI, Camera 1 captured the doctor, Camera 2 all three participants (the doctor, the patient and the interpreter) and Camera 3 the patient. During the remote sessions, the positioning of the three cameras was adapted to allow for a full view of the doctor, the patient and the two of them together, while the interpreter was filmed in the remote location. The display of her screen during VI was captured using XSplit Broadcaster.[3] The

---

3   With the exception of Series 1, during which the screen recording failed for technical reasons.

video cameras used were the Panasonic HC-W850 and the Sony CX700. Backup audio recordings were made of all the sessions with an Edirol R-009 WAV MP3 digital audio/voice recorder. In a next step, the recordings of the different cameras and screen captures were synchronized using the transcription software ELAN to allow for a simultaneous view of the participants from different angles.[4]

4.2.6 Transcription and translation

For the transcriptions of the audiovisual data, Excel spreadsheets were used, which allowed for a quick overview of annotations of the three series and interpreting methods. Figure 3 presents an example of an empty spreadsheet. In these annotation spreadsheets, thirteen categories were noted from left to right: the phase of the consultation (PH); time frame (TIME); number (NR); participant speaking (doctor/patient/interpreter, D/P/I); type of utterance (original utterance, rendition, reactive token, U/R/RT); link (indicating concurrence or non-concurrence); transcript of the original utterance, rendition or reactive token; English gloss; message equivalence issues (ME); interactional issues (IA); repair and optimization strategies (RO); reactive tokens (RT); and environmental and technological issues (ET).

Next to the annotated items, four columns were created to allow for comments on the following categories: message equivalence issues, interactional issues, repair and optimization strategies, and environmental and technological issues.

4 <https://archive.mpi.nl/tla/elan>.

Figure 3. Example of empty annotation spreadsheet.

PH	TIME	NR	D/ P/I	U/R/ ET	Link?	Original utterance/ Rendition/ RT	Gloss	ME	IA	RO	RT	ET	Comment ME	Comment IA	Comment RO	Comment ET

For the transcriptions of the utterances, renditions and reactive tokens, I created my own conventions (see Transcription key) instead of using the widely used transcription conventions proposed by Jefferson (1974), which propose very detailed symbols to describe discourse features such as silences, pitch, emphasis and so on. This choice was guided by the holistic approach adopted in my research, which focuses on examining several phenomena simultaneously (message equivalence issues, interactional dynamics and the influence of environmental and technological factors), and is in line with Gallez's (2022: 55) argument that, traditionally, DI research adopts the detailed CA transcription format, despite its reduced readability when used for multilingual communicative events. In the analyses, I wanted to avoid a granular description of all discourse-analytic features, since not all of these were necessarily relevant to the analysis. However, although prosodic phenomena such as emphasis or intonation were not systematically transcribed, these features were taken into account in the multimodal analyses and were discussed insofar as they were relevant to the analysis.

With regard to the translations of the transcriptions of the audiovisual data (in Dutch and French, the languages used in the simulations) into English, I opted for a pragmatic approach (Hale, 2004: 213) and attempted to remain close to the source text, while at the same time avoiding ungrammatical constructions or non-idiomatic expressions, unless such constructions or expressions were found in the original utterances or renditions. The same approach was followed for the translation of the interviews.

4.3 Annotation

As a first step in preparing the data for analysis, the transcriptions of the video-recorded simulations were annotated. For this purpose, an annotation scheme was designed (Table 7) that aims to identify the most important features related to interpreting quality as discussed in Chapter 3 (miscommunication and interaction management), as well as environmental and technological factors, in order to investigate the impact of the remote conditions, possible relationships between message equivalence issues and interactional issues and the ways in which miscommunication was managed. This resulted in the creation of three main annotation categories:

1. Miscommunication (message equivalence issues and interactional issues)
2. Interaction management (explicit repair and optimization of the communication and backchannelling)
3. Environment and technology

Categories 1 and 2 were both divided into two subcategories. Category 1 (Miscommunication) was subdivided into message equivalence issues and interactional issues. Category 2 (Interaction management) was subdivided into repair and optimization strategies and backchannelling. The typologies of these subcategories were derived top-down on the basis of taxonomies used in empirical research in interpreting studies (Balogh & Hertog, 2012; Baraldi & Gavioli, 2012; Besson et al., 2005; Bot, 2005; Braun, 2004, 2007, 2017; Braun & Taylor, 2012b), medical studies (Flores et al., 2012) and discourse studies (Clancy et al.,1996; Goodwin, 1981; Heritage & Maynard, 2006; Sacks et al., 1974; Schegloff et al., 1977; Whittaker & O'Connaill, 1997; Xudong, 2009; Young & Lee, 2004). These subcategories are discussed in Sections 4.3.1–4.3.3.

Table 7. Annotation model

Miscommunication		Interaction management		Environment & technology
Message equivalence issues	Interactional issues	Repair & optimization	Backchannelling	
Omission	Overlapping speech	Request for clarification	Reactive expression	Operation of equipment
Addition	Pause	Clarification/ Repetition	Resumptive opener	Image quality
Substitution	Language mixing	Meta comment	Repetition	Sound quality
False fluency	Reported speech	Correction	Gaze/Mutual gaze	Connectivity problems
		Compensation	Body posture	Out of shot
		Transformation of reported speech	Gesture	Seating arrangement
		Renditional formulation	Facial expression	Noise
		Change in order	Nod/Head shake	External disturbance

4.3.1 Miscommunication

Message equivalence issues

The annotation model is based on the assumption that there are two parallel levels of communication. The first level is the main level of communication, which is the linguistic content as expressed by the participants, wrapped up in the paralinguistic features (e.g. register, prosody) that give meaning to it. When the source-text content, including its paralinguistic features, was altered or omitted in the rendition in the target text by the interpreter, this was considered an issue at the level of message equivalence. In total, four categories of issues were annotated:

1. Omission: The interpreter omits relevant content-related information or affective elements leading to a loss of important/relevant content;
2. Substitution: The interpreter alters relevant content-related information or affective elements by leaving out an element and adding another one, leading to a change of meaning;
3. Addition: The interpreter adds content-related information or affective elements leading to a change of meaning. When this addition expresses the interpreter's personal opinion, this is referred to as "editorialization" (Flores et al., 2012), which means that interpreters express their own opinion while rendering a participant's message, without the recipient of the message being aware of this. The annotation of editorialization, alongside the linguistic categories, was important to shed light on the interpreter's role and possible changes in that role under different circumstances;
4. False fluency: In the rendition, the interpreter uses either a word/phrase that does not exist in the target language or a completely incorrect word/phrase that substantially alters its meaning (Flores et al., 2012: 546).

Interactional issues

Intertwined with the main level, communication takes place at an interactional level. This level provides a context for the way information is exchanged at the main level. During the interaction between the participants, issues that inhibit smooth communication may arise. These so-called interactional issues can become problematic in interpreter-mediated communication and may be heightened in RI (Braun & Taylor, 2012b). Often, interactional issues occur in combination with each other, for example, a pause leading to overlapping speech. In this category, four items were annotated:

1. Overlapping speech: This occurs when two people speak at the same time and includes both competitive and non-competitive

speech (Shegloff, 2000). While the first type refers to instances in which both participants "fight" to take the floor, the latter includes overlaps that are no attempt to take the floor, such as brief listening responses, indications of understanding or the lack thereof and words of agreement or disagreement (*ibid.*). Overlapping speech does not necessarily mean that a turn transfer will take place; the current speaker can also continue his or her turn. Interpreters, too, are responsible for overlapping speech (Bot, 2005), for example, by starting a rendition while a primary participant has not yet finished his or her turn;

2. Pause: Pauses were annotated when they occurred together with overlapping speech. Following Schegloff et al. (1977), a distinction was made between an intra-turn pause and an inter-turn pause, the first one being a gap or lapse within the turn of a speaker who has the floor, while the latter constitutes a space between two turns. A pause can cause overlapping speech when it is intended as an intra-turn pause by a current speaker, but considered an inter-turn pause by the next speaker, who assumes the current speaker has finished and begins the next turn;
3. Language mixing: The interpreter speaks in two languages within a single turn, which can occur due to confusion and/or cognitive overload;
4. Reported speech: Instead of addressing each other by means of the first and second personal pronoun (I, you), which is encouraged by most codes of ethics, the participants refer to each other by means of the third person (e.g. "he/she", "the doctor", "madame"), using a reporting verb (e.g. "he says") (Bot, 2005).

The last two phenomena (Items 3 and 4) may indicate underlying communication problems and/or cognitive overload, but can also occur as meta comments during explicit repair strategies. When this occurred in the data, these cases were not counted as interactional issues, but were considered being part of the interaction management.

Methodology

4.3.2 Interaction management

Repair and optimization

At the interactional level, all participants are engaged in conversation management by providing each other feedback on the comprehension of the information exchanged at the main level of communication. They do this, firstly, to achieve their communicative goals by optimizing the communication, and prevent miscommunication, for example, by explicitly commenting on the discourse meta structure (e.g. when the doctor announces: "I will now ask you a few short questions, one by one"). Secondly, interaction management can also be aimed at repairing miscommunication, for example, by explicitly requesting clarification. The notion of repair refers to the mechanisms through which certain "troubles" in the interactional dynamics are dealt with (Sacks et al., 1974) and comprises all practices for dealing with problems of hearing, speaking and understanding talk (Schegloff et al., 1977), ranging from turn-taking issues to content-related issues. In interpreter-mediated bilingual conversations, repair mechanisms are even more crucial than in monolingual communication, since the interpreter must continuously attempt to establish a mutual understanding between different participants who speak different languages and have different cultural backgrounds (Bao-Rozée, 2016). In our annotation model, the following strategies for repair and optimization were annotated:

1. Request for clarification: Explicit demand to explain or repeat a certain utterance;
2. Clarification/repetition: Requested or unrequested explanation or repetition of a certain utterance;
3. Meta comment: Comment on the communication process which is not a clarification or a request for clarification, but rather an initiation of a repair (Sacks et al., 1974), comments following repair, or explicit references to the discourse structure (e.g. when a doctor announces that s/he will start by asking a few short questions one by one and will then turn to an in-depth examination);

4. Correction: Explicit or implicit auto-correction of an utterance or a rendition;
5. Compensation: An omission at the level of message equivalence in the same turn or during a previous turn that is implicitly compensated for by means of an addition;
6. Transformation of reported speech: Reported speech (indirect third-person reference) transformed into direct, first-person speech (e.g. the patient's utterance: "Can the doctor tell me …?" is transformed by the interpreter into: "Can you tell me …?");
7. Renditional formulation: The interpreter provides a rendition which is specifically designed to summarize, gloss or develop the gist of one or more previous turns (Baraldi & Gavioli, 2012; Heritage & Maynard, 2006);
8. Change in order: The interpreter changes the chronological order in which the information was provided in the source message, which is often a strategy to cope with complicated information or long turns, for example, by starting the rendition with the end of the speaker's turn, instead of the beginning.

Items 1–3 can be used by all participants, whereas Items 4–8 are exclusively used by the interpreter in his or her renditions of source-text utterances.

Backchannelling

Besides repair and optimization strategies, the signalling of comprehension or non-comprehension – as well as agreement or non-agreement with an utterance by another speaker – can also be expressed less explicitly (e.g. by using facial expressions). We will refer to this part of the interaction management as "backchannelling", that is, behaviour by means of which speakers and listeners derive key information to clarify content and provide feedback (Whittaker & O'Connaill, 1997: 28–29). Backchannelling behaviour is also referred to as "reactive tokens" (Clancy et al., 1996; Young & Lee, 2004), or "response tokens" (Gardner, 2001) and can be visual, verbal or a combination of the two. Backchannelling helps speakers and listeners coordinate their content accordingly

(Goodwin, 1981) and can also help maintain the smooth flow of communication (Roy, 2000). The analysis of visible aspects such as gaze, posture and gesture provides insight into the communicative meaning of participants' actions (Krystallidou, 2016; Vranjes, 2018), as well as into their engagement in the interaction (Goodwin, 1981). Moreover, the sequential timing of backchannels is important, since by providing particular feedback at a particular point in the interaction, addressees can actively steer the interaction in a particular direction (Tolins & Fox Tree, 2014).

For this category, the following eight items were annotated:

1. Reactive expression: Short, non-floor-taking, lexical or non-lexical vocalizations (e.g. "oh"), reactive phrases ("that's great") or words ("all right"), produced by the listener, serving as a display of attention, interest, claim of understanding or acknowledgement (Xudong, 2009);
2. Resumptive opener: Specific type of non-lexical or lexical reactive expression that, in a sequential context, serves to acknowledge the prior turn and indicate a new turn (*ibid.*). There is normally a short pause between a resumptive opener and the full turn following it;
3. Repetition: Type of lexical reactive expression acknowledging what the previous speaker has said by repeating the speaker's word(s);
4. Gaze/mutual gaze: Gaze is an important communicative signal to demonstrate attention and engagement, and to manage turn-taking between the participants (Bavelas et al., 2002; Goodwin, 1981; Kendon, 1967). Whereas in natural conversations, listeners usually direct their gaze towards the speaker and vice versa (when this happens simultaneously, this is called mutual gaze or "gaze window" [Bavelas et al., 2002]), in interpreter-mediated conversations, the primary participants are encouraged to look at each other and not at the interpreter (Bot, 2005);
5. Body posture: More or less stable state of the body, not to be confused with gestures, since these imply movement (Besson et al., 2005);

6. Gesture: Used to manage turn transfer and accompany speech. Gestures can encourage or discourage a person to speak or continue (Bot, 2005: 130). In healthcare interpreting specifically, gesturing is also used to convey information on physical symptoms (Gerwing & Li, 2019);
7. Facial expression: Dynamic features which communicate speakers' and listeners' attitudes, emotions and intentions, such as smiling, frowning or yawning (Besson et al., 2005). Facial expressions play an important role in making sense of the reception or intention of a message and can resolve potential ambiguities (Braun, 2012);
8. Nod/Head shake: Used to acknowledge, agree or disagree in a nonverbal manner.

4.3.3 Environment and technology

Together, the main level and the interactional level of communication form a subtle verbal and nonverbal interplay between listener and speaker, who constantly exchange turns following a certain turn-taking pattern, in line with the discourse context. The two levels can affect each other and can, in turn, be directly or indirectly influenced by contextual factors that affect smooth communication, such as environmental or technological conditions. The annotation category Environment and technology (ET) consists of the following eight items:

1. Equipment: Operation of the RI devices, for example, adjusting the volume of the telephone or the position of the webcam for appropriate sound or view, or the act of reconnecting in case of a technical breakdown;
2. Image quality: Blurry or frozen image;
3. Sound quality: Reduced volume or sound distortion;
4. Connectivity problems: Loss or partial loss of the internet connection (during VI);
5. Out of shot: Being within the field of the camera or not (during VI);

Methodology

6. Seating: The way the participants position themselves in the space, for example, in a triadic constellation during F2FI;
7. Noise: Any sound that may compromise audibility between the participants;
8. Other external disturbances: For example, an unauthorized person entering the recording room.

4.4 Analysis

In this section, I explain how the annotated data were analysed. First, the different phases in medical consultations are described (Section 4.4.1). Subsequently, the units of analysis are explained (Section 4.4.2). After that, I explain how potential relationships between issues at the levels of message equivalence and interaction were investigated by elaborating on the concept of concurrence (Section 4.4.3). Lastly, Section 4.4.4 describes how the interview data were processed.

4.4.1 *Phases in the consultation*

The structure of doctor–patient consultations can be divided into five genre steps: (1) opening phase, (2) problem presentation, (3) verbal and/or physical examination, (4) diagnosis, treatment and check-ups, and (5) closing (based on Byrne & Long, 1984/1976; Heritage & Maynard, 2006). The structure of follow-up visits are often less structured (Heritage & Maynard, 2006), as was the case in some of the consultations that were simulated for the current research.

Following the example of Amato (2018), the five genre steps were reduced to three main parts ("introduction", "body" and "closing"). However, since issues such as overlapping speech are potentially more problematic when they occur during the body of the consultation (where they may lead to the omission of important content) than when they happen during the introductory or closing phase, only the bodies of the simulations – consisting of the presentation of the complaints, examination and treatment – were annotated. The management of the opening and closing phases from the consultations in each series were analysed separately. Since openings and closings are of major importance in establishing rapport between the participants, as demonstrated in research on monolingual healthcare communication (Heath, 2004/1986) and interpreter-mediated communication (Braun & Davitti, 2018), contextualizing actions and utterances in these phases is an essential part of assessing the quality of interpreter-mediated communication. Moreover, as Braun and Davitti (2018) argue, previous research has demonstrated that opening and closing phases of conversations are more challenging in RI than in F2FI.

4.4.2 Units of analysis

As explained in Chapter 3, this research conceptualizes interpreter-mediated medical consultations as triadic conversations that take place within a specific institutional discourse framework and consist of content that is continuously co-constructed and negotiated by all three parties (healthcare provider, patient, interpreter). Within this discourse framework, the communication is organized sequentially with turns, which are the units on which the qualitative analyses are based. According to Conversation Analysis, turns consist of turn-constructional units (TCU's), which are the grammatical units with which a speaker may construct a turn. They have also been described as the "building blocks" that constitute turns (Sidnell, 2009: 21). TCU's include sentences, clauses, phrases or single words (Sacks et al., 1974). In this work, a further distinction is made between full turns (turns that are expressed by a speaker who has the floor) and reactive tokens, that is, non-floor taking responses by a speaker during or immediately following another speaker's turn (Clancy et al., 1996; Young & Lee, 2004). To avoid a distorted comparison of the average turn length as a result of differences in the use of reactive tokens, only full turns (i.e. turns in which one person has the floor as a speaker) were counted to calculate the average turn length in the quantitative analyses. A full turn can consist of the following four units or combinations thereof:

Methodology

1. Original utterance by one of the primary speakers (doctor or patient);
2. Rendition by the interpreter, that is, a translation of a primary speaker's original utterance;
3. "Non-rendition" (Wadensjö, 1998), that is, an original utterance by the interpreter that is not a rendition, but which is expressed on the interpreter's own behalf, for example, an initiation of repair;
4. Combination of an original utterance and a rendition, expressed by the interpreter in one turn. This combination can occur, for example, when the interpreter requests or provides a clarification, or makes a remark on her own behalf during a rendition, while holding the floor.

Each turn is part of a turn-taking pattern following a sequential organization, which proceeds through a recursive chain of interlinked adjacency pairs (Sacks et al., 1974). In medical consultations, this structure gives rise to characteristic three-part sequences of question–response–acknowledgement (Merlini & Favaron, 2007; Mishler, 1984; Silverman, 1987). By initiating questions, the doctor controls the turn-taking system, that is, the way talking turns are distributed between participants (Merlini & Favaron, 2007: 106–108). In interpreter-mediated consultations, the doctor must yield a part of this control to the interpreter (Pasquandrea, 2012: 456), who has his or her turn after every one of these parts in the sequence, thus creating an "adjacency trio" (Merlini & Favaron, 2007: 108). This is called "regular turn-taking" (Roy, 2000: 72).

In the qualitative analyses, the occurrence of miscommunication was studied beyond the units of single turns by looking into sequences of interaction, that is, multiple, interlinked turns following each other and dealing with the same subtopic. An example of such a sequence is as follows: the doctor asks a question – the interpreter renders this question – the patient answers – the interpreter renders the answer.

In the analysis of the sequences, backchannelling signals giving meaning to the content were also taken into account to study the achievement of a mutual understanding between the participants. To reconstruct miscommunication, observed instances of concurrence (i.e. issues occurring at several levels at the same time) were submitted to qualitative analyses.

By means of illustrative excerpts taken from the corpus of audiovisual data, the analyses demonstrate how miscommunication occurred, what caused it and how the interaction was managed across the three different interpreting methods. Following, among others, Davitti (2013) and Davitti and Pasquandrea (2017), in this work, the scope of traditional conversation analysis is broadened to include the study of multimodal aspects of the communication, that is, the ways in which the participants employed the different communicative resources available to them (speech, gesture, gaze, etc.) in the interaction. As Pasquandrea (2011: 456) puts forward, research on DI can particularly benefit from multimodal analysis since it constitutes much more than a simple linguistic transfer, but must be considered a "complex participation format that is likely to be managed multimodally". Especially when using modes of interpreting in which visual access is reduced or altogether absent – as is the case in RI –, multimodal analysis can help demonstrate the ways in which embodied resources are used in these conditions, as well as their efficiency. Multimodal analysis comparing the functioning of the different communication resources under different conditions (with full visual access, reduced access and no access) can shed light on potential differences in interaction management. Therefore, in the discourse-based interactional analyses that are central to the current study, the multimodal nature of human communication – that is, the multitude of communication modes (visual, spoken, gestural, etc.) that contribute to the meaning of message content (Jewitt, 2009) – is taken into account. Insight into these communication features of the collected video data was provided by synchronizing the different camera and screen recordings in ELAN (as explained in Section 4.2.6), which allowed for a very close examination of the participants' multimodal behaviour from different angles.

4.4.3 Concurrence

Identification of problematic issues

After all issues at the levels of message equivalence (ME) and interaction (IA) had been annotated, they were submitted to a quantitative analysis.

It must be stressed that, given the small size of the corpus, the purpose of the quantitative analyses was not to proceed with hypothesis testing or generate statistics, but to identify problematic issues and allow for a qualitative examination of relationships between issues concurring at the different communication levels.

At the ME level, all annotated issues were scrutinized and categorized as *problematic* issues if they led to loss of information, change of meaning or loss of empathic and emotional meaning. In research on TI, omissions of this type are referred to as "unjustifiable omissions" (Wang & Fang, 2019: 45). The reasoning behind the decision to make a distinction between problematic and non-problematic issues was that, if all issues in the ME category, such as omission, were considered inaccuracies at the level of single turns or adjacency pairs (question–answer pairs), the complex interactional process of achieving a mutual understanding through verbal and nonverbal resources and by coordinating activities would be overlooked (Baker, 2006). As Napier (2004: 117) explains, omission can very well be a deliberate linguistic strategy for coping with the direct discourse context and is not necessarily problematic.

ME issues were considered problematic when they caused a loss of important (medical) content, given that this could obviously have serious consequences for the patient's health (Flores et al., 2012). Moreover, renditions leading to a loss of transfer of empathy in the doctor's responses and the patient's expression of emotion, as well as references to patient participation, were considered problematic, since expressions of emotions and empathy are considered crucial to rapport-building between the doctor and the patient and because patient participation is nowadays regarded as an important element of healthcare (Baraldi & Gavioli, 2007; Krystallidou, 2014). As Baraldi and Gavioli (2007: 157) put forward, emotional expressions by the patient, as well as the doctor's affective involvement in the interaction are considered essential in a patient-centred approach.

However, it must be noted that the assessment of the problematic nature of the annotated issues was not always clear-cut and involved a certain degree of subjectivity, especially since, given the limited size of this research project, there was only one rater (the researcher). In cases of doubt about whether a certain issue was to be considered problematic or not, the video recordings of the moment in which a particular instance occurred were thoroughly re-examined, as were the turns preceding and following this instance.

Excerpt 1 illustrates the difference between a non-problematic and problematic ME issue. In all excerpts, the first column shows the turn number from the original annotation sheet and the abbreviations of the issues observed, the second column presents the transcripts of the original utterances, reactive tokens and renditions, and the third column provides the English gloss. The issues observed are marked in bold in the transcripts.

EXAMPLE OF NON-PROBLEMATIC AND PROBLEMATIC ME ISSUES

Excerpt 1 was taken from the F2FI session of Series 1, which dealt with the theme weak pelvic floor.

Excerpt 1. Example of problematic and non-problematic ME issues

| 79 | D: […] daar geef ik de papieren voor mee, **dan kunt u bij het laboratorium urine inleveren**, krijgt u bij de balie de vragenlijsten, verwijs ik u naar de fysiotherapeut en als u daar de intake hebt gehad en dat loopt, komt u nog een keer terug **om de uitslag samen te bespreken.** | D: […] for that I will give you the papers **then you can hand in urine at the laboratory**, you will receive the questionnaires at the desk, I direct you towards the physical therapist and when you will have had your intake there and it's running, you will return once more to me **to discuss the results together.** |
| 80 OM SUB | I: Euh, je vais vous donner un papier pour **aller au laboratoire**. Vous pouvez chercher à l'accueil également le questionnaire pour le compléter. Je vais prescrire la physiothérapie. Et puis je vais vous demander après un certain temps de revenir vers moi, **on va voir comment tout se passe.** | I: Euh, I am going to give you a paper to go **to the laboratory**. You can also go to the desk for the questionnaire to complete it. I am going to prescribe the physiotherapy. And also I am also going to ask you after a certain time to come back to me, **we are going to see how everything is going**. |

Note: D = doctor, I = interpreter, OM = omission, SUB = substitution.
For further details of the transcription conventions, see Transcription key.

Methodology

In Excerpt 1, the interpreter (I) omits (OM, Turn 80) a part of the instructions provided by the doctor (D) in Turn 78, that is, the fact that the patient (P) has to hand in a urine sample at the laboratory. Since this had been discussed earlier in the consultation, there is little risk of a possible misunderstanding. Therefore, this omission was considered non-problematic. However, within the same rendition (Turn 80), the interpreter produces a substitution (SUB). The doctor's utterance that they will "discuss the results together" (Turn 79) is rendered by the interpreter as "we are going to see how everything is going" (Turn 80). This substitution (SUB) is considered problematic, since the explicit reference to patient participation through the doctor's use of "together" is lost in the interpreter's rendition.

An inventory was also made of all annotated issues at the IA level. When several IA issues were directly linked to each other (e.g. a pause leading to overlapping speech), these were considered one cluster of IA issues. At the IA level, it was not possible to make a quantitative selection of problematic issues, since their potential problematic nature was much more difficult to establish without further analysis of the complete sequence than was the case for ME issues. Whether the annotated IA issues were in fact problematic or not depended on their concurrence with ME or ET issues. This will be further explained in the next section (Identification of concurrence).

With regard to the interaction management, an account was made of the strategies to repair miscommunication and optimize communication in order to establish how much of the communication was dedicated to repair and to speech acts other than translating. These quantitative results were compared across the three interpreting methods.

Identification of concurrence

To investigate the causes of miscommunication, a quantitative analysis of all annotated issues at the levels of message equivalence (ME) and interaction (IA) was conducted, and an inventory produced of issues related to environment and technology (ET). To examine the relationships between these different categories of issues, I studied their concurrence, that is, their simultaneous occurrence.

First, a distinction was made between issues that happened independently from issues in other categories ("non-concurrences") and those that happened in conjunction with issues from different categories (ME, IA, ET) ("concurrences"). Secondly, I examined the cases of concurrence to verify if a relationship between the issues concurring in two or more categories could be observed, and, in case issues from the ET category were involved, what role the environmental and technological factors played in the concurrence of the ME and IA issues.

Subsequently, in the qualitative analyses of each series, the cases of concurrence were studied and compared across the interpreting methods. Following Heath (2004/1986: 7), these micro-analyses took contextual aspects into account, that is, "the location of the investigated action in a phased activity within the encounter" as well as "their placement in a specific and autochthonously intelligible sequence and course of action" that give meaning to the utterances and actions under investigation. Moreover, the micro-analyses of the sequences involving concurrence consider the ways in which verbal and nonverbal resources were combined in the management of the interaction.

To illustrate the difference between cases of concurrence and non-concurrence, I will provide two examples. The first example (Excerpt 2) demonstrates a case in which issues concurred at different levels, but after closer examination, turned out not be related. The second example (Excerpt 3) illustrates a case of concurrence where, after closer examination, a relationship between issues at different levels was established.

EXAMPLE OF NON-CONCURRENCE

Excerpt 2 was taken from the VI session of Series 1 (VI-1), which dealt with heavy menstrual bleeding. The doctor has suggested an IUD to mitigate the patient's complaints, after which the patient wants to know more about the effects of the IUD.

Methodology

Excerpt 2. Example of non-related concurring issues (VI-1)

47	P: [...] J'ai l'impression que ... oui, je sais pas, après que c'est sûr que je puisse avoir euh facilement des enfants ? Euh je ne sais pas, stérilet, **ça fait un peu peur, on dit que ça peut faire très mal, quand on n'a pas des enfants et après, euh ...**	P: [...] I have the impression that ... well, I don't know, after that is it sure that I can euh easily have children? Euh I don't know, IUD, **it scares me a bit, they say it can hurt a lot, when you don't have children and after, euh ...**
48 SQ OM FF	I: [...] En ja, ik het gehoord dat het eigenlijk pijnlijk is als je kinderwens niet vervuld is.	I [...] And well, I have heard that it's in fact painful when your desire to have children is not fulfilled.
49 RCL	D: Kunt u dat laatste nog eens herhalen, want daar stoorde het een beetje.	D: Could you repeat the last thing, because there was some disturbance.
50 META CLA/ REP RS	I: Euhm, van het moment dat, ja, vanaf mevrouw zei **mevrouw vraagt bent u zeker dat ik nog kinderen zal**	I: Euhm, from the moment that, yes madam said **madam asks are you sure that I can still have children**
51 OS	D: **Vanaf ...** **vanaf** dat het pijnlijk is	D: **From ... from** that it is painful
50	I: kunnen krijgen, achteraf kinderen zal kunnen krijgen euhm, want ik heb gehoord dat het pijnlijk is als u dat niet kunt, als je kinderwens niet vervuld is.	I: have children afterwards euhm, because I have heard that is painful when you can't, if your desire to have children has not been fulfilled.

Note: P = patient, I = interpreter, D = doctor, SQ = sound quality, OM = omission, FF = false fluency, RCL = request for clarification, META = meta comment, CLA/REP = clarification/repetition, OS = overlapping speech. For further details of the transcription conventions see Transcription key

In Turn 47, the patient says she is worried she might not be able to have children after the IUD and that she is somewhat scared about the IUD, because "they say that it can hurt a lot when you don't have children", indicating that she is afraid that it may be painful to have the IUD placed when one has not given birth yet. The interpreter omits the utterance "it scares me a bit" (OM) and misunderstands the patient's message: She produces a false fluency (FF) by rendering the content as follows: "I have heard that it is painful when your desire to have children has not been fulfilled" (Turn 48). At that moment, there is a problem with the sound quality (SQ), which prompts the doctor to request clarification (RCL, Turn 49). The interpreter clarifies the matter by repeating the false fluency (CLA/REP, Turn 50). During the repair, there is overlapping speech (OS) with the doctor (Turn 51). In this example, the deterioration of the sound quality leads to repair and overlapping speech, but has no relationship with the occurring ME issues (omission, false fluency) in the rendition. Therefore, the combination of the ET issue and ME issue in this sequence was considered a case of non-concurrence.

Example of concurrence

Excerpt 3 was taken from the last phase of the consultation in the same session (VI-1), just before the closing.

Excerpt 3. Example of related concurring issues (VI-1)

125 N SQ	P: D'accord, c'est bien, ça me paraît bien. Puis, oui, tant qu'on peut l'enlever, moi, ça va. (..) Voilà. Mais de toute façon, il faut bien essayer quelque chose parce que c'est tuant ce truc de règles, j'en ai marre.	P: Okay, it's fine, that looks good to me. Also, well, as long as you can remove it, for me it's okay. (..) So. But in any case, we must try something because it's killing me this period thing, I am fed up with it.
126 RCL	I: J'ai pas compris pas la dernière **phrase.**	I: I did not understand the last **phrase.**
127 META CLA	P: **J'ai dit il** faut bien essayer quelque chose parce que ça me ... j'en peux plus de ce truc de règles, donc euh, voilà. Il faut essayer quelque chose.	P: **I said that** we have to do something because it's.. I am fed up with this period thing, so euh, that's it. We have to try something.

Methodology

Excerpt 3. Continued

| 128 | I: Euhm, pff, ja dat lijkt me goed, vooral als ik weet dat het spiraaltje verwijderd kan worden zeker. Want de regels, de menstruatie da da da ben kiek beu. | I: Euhm, pff, yes, that looks good to me, especially if I know that the IUD can be removed for sure. Because these periods, this menstruation tha tha that I am fed up with. |

Note: D = doctor, I = interpreter, N/SQ = noise/sound quality, RCL = request for clarification, META = meta comment, CLA = clarification. For further details of the transcription conventions see Transcription key

The patient says she is fine with having the IUD placed and expresses her anxiety about solving the problem she has (heavy periods), by saying, "it's killing me this period thing" (Turn 125). During this turn, there is noise (N) in the consultation room, which causes sound quality (SQ) problems for the interpreter, who informs the patient that she has not understood the last phrase by means of a request for clarification (RCL, Turn 126). The patient (Turn 127) only partly repeats what she has said in her previous turn and leaves out the part "it's killing me". Since this was exactly the part that the interpreter did not hear because of the sound quality problem, we can conclude that the environmental/technological problem had a direct effect on omission (OM) in the form of loss of message content. Therefore, the combination of the ET issue and the ME issue was considered a case of concurrence.

4.4.4 Interview data

As a final step in the process of the data analysis, the results of the objective quality assessment were triangulated with the participants' perceptions, collected in post-simulation interviews. These consisted of short, semi-structured interviews with all participants immediately after the simulations and in-depth interviews with the interpreters two weeks after the simulations, once a first, basic analysis of the simulation video data had been done.

After each simulation, all three participants (doctor, simulated patient, interpreter) answered questions during semi-structured interviews conducted by the researcher. In these short interviews – which took approximately 5 minutes per person – each participant was questioned individually about her satisfaction with the communication, the quality of care and the interpreting, the technical conditions and the seating arrangement, as well as about her preferences with regard to the different interpreting methods. The purpose of these short interviews was to complement the objective analyses of the simulation video data and determine to what extent the subjective and objective assessments of the communication quality aspects corresponded to one another. Two weeks after each series, the interpreters were interviewed once more to comment on specific issues that had come up during the researcher's initial analysis. These in-depth interviews had the objective of contextualizing salient aspects of the interpreters' behaviour and to complement and verify the accuracy of certain observations (Maxwell, 2013). The average duration of these interviews was around 15 minutes.

All interview data – a total of thirty interviews, that is, twenty-seven short, semi-structured interviews and three in-depth interviews – were transcribed and translated from French and Dutch into English. Subsequently, the participants' perceptions of the quality aspects mentioned above were compared and linked to the findings from the objective quality analysis of the video data. The data collected from the in-depth interviews with the interpreters were analysed in order to identify overarching themes and used to put into perspective certain observations in the discussion of the results from the qualitative analyses of the simulations.

The following part (Part III) presents and discusses the results from the data analysis. It starts with an overview of miscommunication, interaction management and concurrence in Chapter 5. Subsequently, it moves on to looker deeper into the specific challenges to communication quality in Chapter 6, as observed in the simulations. These challenges are triangulated by the results from the participant perception of communication quality in Chapter 7, collected by means of the interviews. The overall results across the series come together in the discussion of the main conclusions in Chapter 8, in which I will also discuss implications of the research results for interpreting training and practice. Part III finishes with a brief outline of the limitations of this study and directions for future research.

PART III
Results

CHAPTER 5

Miscommunication and Interaction Management

In this chapter, I present the results of the analysis of ME and IA issues, and, by looking into concurrence, discuss to what extent relationships between issues at different levels were established. As explained in Section 4.3, miscommunication was defined as the occurrence of issues at one or both of the intertwined communication levels, that is, the level of message equivalence (ME) and of interaction (IA). ME issues were defined as issues that occurred at the main level of communication and concerned instances in which the source-text content, including its paralinguistic features, was altered or omitted in the interpreter's target-text rendition. IA issues were defined as issues that inhibited smooth communication at the interactional level. Interaction management refers to the ways in which participants organize their interaction, including how they deal with and prevent miscommunication.

This chapter starts with a quantitative comparison of miscommunication across the three series and interpreting methods by looking into numbers, types and examples of miscommunication at the levels of message equivalence (Section 5.1) and interaction (Section 5.2). Subsequently, in order to identify potential relationships between the categories of issues, an inventory of the interaction management (consisting of repair and optimization strategies) is made (Section 5.3), as well as of instances of concurrence (Section 5.4). These quantitative analyses provide the basis for the qualitative analysis of specific challenges at the level of miscommunication and interaction management discussed in Chapter 6.

5.1 Message equivalence issues

In this category, four types of issues were annotated: omission, substitution, addition and false fluency (Table 7).

5.1.1 Frequency of ME issues

To fully grasp the results for the ME issues, the calculation for the frequency of issues must first be clarified. To allow for a more natural interaction (Section 4.2.3), non-scripted scenarios were used for the simulations. As a result, the simulated consultations varied in their total duration. In order to compare the frequency of issues across the simulations, we normalized the simulation duration based on the average (1,250 seconds). In this way, the number of issues occurring per 1,250 seconds were calculated. A disadvantage of this calculation is that it does not take into account the possible gradual increase in issues throughout the simulations as a result of cognitive overload, as demonstrated by, for example, Braun (2013). However, the progression of problematic issues in the course of each simulation is discussed in the qualitative analyses.

Table 8 indicates the frequency of problematic ME issues in Series 1, 2 and 3 for the three interpreting methods (F2FI, TI and VI). This was calculated by multiplying the number of issues by the average duration of all nine simulations (1,250 seconds). The resulting product was then divided by the total duration of the simulation in question in seconds. For example, in the F2FI session in Series 1, the absolute ("abs") number of problematic ME issues was thirty-three. The duration of this simulation was 23 minutes and 59 seconds (Table 3), that is, 1,439 seconds, while the average duration of the simulations was 1,250 seconds. This was calculated as: 33 (absolute number of issues) × 1,250 (average simulation duration in seconds) / 1,439 (duration in seconds of the simulation in question) = 28.66. In a last step, this outcome was rounded off to 28.7, which is the relative ("rel") number of issues in the F2FI session in Series 1. The descriptive analyses will refer to the relative numbers.

Table 8. Frequency of message equivalence issues

	Interpreting method						Total	
	F2FI		TI		VI			
	abs	rel	abs	rel	abs	rel	abs	rel
Series 1	33	28.7	37	26.1	33	27.5	103	82.3
Series 2	42	42.0	33	41.3	66	54.0	141	137.3
Series 3	16	21.7	26	34.7	08	11.2	50	67.6

Note. abs = absolute frequency, rel = relative frequency

Table 8 shows that, in terms of the number of problematic ME issues in the performance of each interpreter for each method, no clear patterns across the interpreting methods can be observed.

The performance of Interpreter 1 was the most regular, with only a few differences in the number of issues across the interpreting methods (F2FI: 28.7; TI: 26.1; VI: 27.5). Obviously, in Series 1, the remote conditions had little effect on the number of ME issues.

In Series 2 and 3, the differences in performance at the ME level across the three interpreting methods were greater, but no similar patterns were observed between the two series. In Series 2, a relatively high number of ME issues occurred in VI (54.0) compared with F2FI (42.0) and TI (41.3). By contrast, in Series 3, the number of ME issues was clearly lower in VI (11.2) than in F2FI (21.7), and highest in TI (34.7).

As far as the total number of ME issues per series (and therefore per interpreter) is concerned, a large gap can be observed between Series 1 (82.3) and Series 3 (67.6) on the one hand, and Series 2 (137.3) on the other. Despite the fact that all three interpreters met the strict selection criteria explained in Section 4.2.2, Interpreter 2 produced more than 1.5 times as many problematic ME issues as Interpreter 1, and even twice as many as Interpreter 3. These results suggest that the individual competence of the interpreters had a strong influence on the interpreting quality at the ME level.

5.1.2 Types of ME issues

Table 9 shows the frequency of the different types of message equivalence (ME) issues in Series 1, 2 and 3 across the three interpreting methods. For each series and interpreting method, the absolute frequency, the relative frequency (i.e. the normalized frequency) and the percentage of the types of issues based on the total number of problematic ME issues are provided. For the sake of clarity, the percentages for the subcategories were rounded off to one decimal place, whereas the total numbers were rounded off to 100.

Table 9. Types of message equivalence issues

	Series 1			Series 2			Series 3		
	abs	rel	%	abs	rel	%	abs	rel	%
F2FI									
Omission	19	16.5	57.6	27	27.0	64.3	8	10.9	50.0
Addition	1	0.9	3.0	2	2.0	4.8	n.p.	n.p.	n.p.
Substitution	7	6.1	21.2	10	10.0	23.9	6	8.1	37.5
False fluency	6	5.2	18.2	3	3.0	7.1	2	2.7	12.5
Total F2FI	33	28.7	100	42	42.0	100	16	21.7	100
TI									
Omission	20	14.1	54.1	18	22.5	54.6	16	21.3	61.5
Addition	3	2.1	08.1	2	2.5	0.6	1	01.4	03.8
Substitution	3	9.2	35.1	9	11.3	27.3	6	08.0	23.0
False fluency	1	0.7	02.7	4	5.0	12.1	3	04.0	11.5
Total TI	37	26.1	100	33	41.3	100	26	34.7	100
VI									
Omission	20	16.7	60.6	30	24.6	45.5	7	9.8	87.5
Addition	2	1.7	6.1	9	7.4	13.7	n.p.	n.p.	n.p.
Substitution	4	3.4	12.1	13	10.7	19.7	n.p.	n.p.	n.p.
False fluency	7	5.8	21.2	14	11.5	21.1	1	1.4	12.5
Total VI	33	27.5	100	66	54.0	100	8	11.2	100

Note. abs = absolute frequency, rel = relative frequency, n.p. = not present

Table 9 shows that, across the series and interpreting methods, omission was the prevailing type of ME issue, ranging from 45.5 per cent (Series 2) up to 87.5 per cent (Series 3). As far as the other types of ME issues are concerned (addition, substitution, false fluency), no comparable patterns were observed across the three series. Within each individual series, the lowest variation in types of ME issues was observed in Series 1, whereas the highest variation occurred in Series 3. However, as the relative numbers indicate, it must be borne in mind that in Series 3, the total number of omissions was three times lower than in Series 2. The variations in numbers and types of ME issues will be discussed in more detail in the qualitative analysis of the simulations in the following chapters.

Possible impact of the simulation order

As explained in Section 4.2.3, in each series, the simulations were carried out in a different order. This was based on the results of previous remote interpreting studies, especially on VI (Braun, 2004, 2007; Braun & Taylor, 2012b; Balogh & Hertog, 2012; Balogh & Salaets, 2018), which indicate that in the course of an interpreter-mediated event, the number of errors increased more rapidly in RI conditions than in F2FI conditions.

Table 10 shows the chronological order in which the simulations were performed (1st, 2nd and 3rd) and the number of ME issues that occurred in each series, for each method. For example, in Series 1, the first simulation was F2FI, the second one VI and the third TI.

Table 10. Order of interpreting method vs number of message equivalence issues

	1st	rel	2nd	rel	3rd	rel
Series 1	F2FI	28.7	VI	27.5	TI	26.1
Series 2	TI	42.0	F2FI	41.3	VI	54.0
Series 3	VI	11.2	TI	34.7	F2FI	21.7

Note. rel = relative number of message equivalence issues

Table 10 shows that, on the one hand, in Series 1, there were hardly any differences in numbers between the interpreting methods. On the other hand, in Series 2 and 3, there were large discrepancies in the number of ME issues between the interpreting methods. However, in Series 2, the highest number of issues occurred during the last simulation, whereas in Series 3, it was in the second simulation. Based on these observations, no direct link between the number of ME issues and the chronological order of the simulations could be established.

5.1.3 *Examples of ME issues*

The ME issues presented below were observed in all nine simulations and include problematic, non-concurring issues. As explained in Section 4.4.3 within the two categories of issues (ME issues and IA issues), a distinction was made between issues which occurred independently from issues in other categories ("non-concurrences") and issues which concurred in conjunction with issues in both the ME category and IA category and/or in the category of environmental/technological issues ("concurrences"). Subsequently, cases of concurrence were examined to establish if there was indeed a relationship between the concurring issues. These will be analysed in Chapter 6.

Excerpts 4–12 here illustrate different types of ME issues (omission, addition, substitution, false fluency, or a combination thereof) that were observed in the complete corpus of simulations. They were categorized as problematic for the following reasons:

1. Important or specific content regarding the treatment/procedure or nuances mitigating the message are left out (omission, Example 1a and 1b), strengthened (substitution, Example 1c) or transferred incorrectly (false fluency, Example 1d);
2. Omission of reference to patient participation or patient empowerment (Example 2);
3. Substitution of specific medical terminology (Example 3);
4. Omission of expression of empathy (Example 4);

5. Omission of expression of emotions and anxiety (Example 5);
  6. Editorialization (the interpreter adds her own opinion, Example 6).

As explained, three interpreters participated in the simulation. Throughout the analyses, the interpreters performing in Series 1, 2 and 3 will be referred to as "Interpreter 1", "Interpreter 2" and "Interpreter 3", respectively. In the analysis of the excerpts, the interpreter is referred to as "the interpreter" (I), while the primary participants (the doctor and the patient) are called "the doctor" (D) and "the patient" (P). In each of the excerpts, the first column gives the turn/rendition number. In the next two columns, the left one shows the original utterances by the doctor (D) or patient (P) and the renditions by the interpreter (I), whereas the column on the right provides an English gloss. The top row shows the interpreting method (F2FI, VI, or TI) as well as the series number from which the excerpt was taken (Series 1, 2 or 3). For example, F2FI-1 refers to the simulation using face-to-face interpreting in Series 1.

The video data were transcribed in a simplified way compared with the generally used Jeffersonian transcription conventions (Section 4.2.6). This choice was guided by the holistic approach of this research, which examines several phenomena at the same time (message equivalence issues, interactional issues and the influence of environmental and technological factors) and illustrates these with significant examples. To maintain an overview of the phenomena across the three series, a granular description of all discourse-analytic features in the examples was avoided. Nevertheless, specific multimodal features were taken into account in the analyses insofar as they were relevant to the qualitative analysis.

With respect to glossing the transcriptions (which are originally in Dutch and French, the languages used in the simulations) in English, I opted for a pragmatic approach (Hale, 2004), rather than a literal (word-for-word) or semantic (sentence-by-sentence) approach. Further details concerning this choice are explained in Section 4.2.6.

Excerpt 4. (F2FI-1)

| 69 | D: Dat gaat **in 90 procent van de gevallen** een **hele grote** verbetering opleveren. | D: That will give, **in 90 per cent of the cases**, a **very big** improvement. |
| 70 OM OM | I: Je prévois de l'amélioration avec cela. | I: I expect improvement with that. |

1a. Omission of specific information from the doctor regarding treatment

In the example presented in Excerpt 4, specific information from the doctor in Turn 69 about the efficiency of the proposed treatment – that is, that "in 90 per cent of the cases" the treatment will lead to "a very big improvement" of the patient's situation – is omitted (OM), as is the doctor's reassurance that the improvement is expected to be "very big" (Turn 69).

1b. Omission of nuances of the doctor's message content makes the rendition stronger than the original utterance

Excerpt 5. (F2FI-3)

| 47 | D: Euhm, want in het vorige gesprek hebben we het gehad over euh uw voorgeschiedenis, medicijnen en wat u daar onder andere heeft verteld is **dat u euh euhm regelmatig alcohol drinkt en soms ook weleens drugs gebruikt.** | D: Ehm, because in the previous conversation we talked about eh your anamnesis, medication and what you said then among other things is that you eh ehm drink alcohol **regularly** and **sometimes** use drugs **from time to time**. |
| 48 OM OM | I: Oui, parce que dans l'entretien précédent on a parlé de votre passé hein, donc euh euh les médicaments que vous preniez et cétéra donc euh, dans cet entretien vous avez signalé aussi que vous (..) consommiez de l'alcool et que vous aviez aussi consommé de la drogue. | I: Yes, because in the previous conversation we talked about your past aye, so eh eh the medication that you were taking et cetera so eh, in that conversation you reported also that you (..) consumed alcohol and that you had also consumed drugs. |

In Excerpt 5, the doctor reminds the patient that in a previous consultation, they discussed the patient's habits concerning the use of drugs and alcohol (Turn 47). By omitting the nuances "regularly", "sometimes" and the repetition "from time to time" when referring to these drinking and drug-use habits (OM, Turn 48), Interpreter 3 renders the doctor's rather soft and gentle way of dealing with this delicate subject in a less empathic and more straightforward way. The interpreter's pause, transcribed as "(…)", indicates a moment of hesitation where the interpreter apparently briefly thinks of a way to formulate the rendition and does not immediately find an equivalent way of expressing the nuances of the original utterance.

1c. Substitution: The rendition is less specific than the original utterance

Excerpt 6. (F2FI-2)

26	D: Euhm, **met het effect van yoga of acupunctuur op deze klachten** heb ik geen ervaring […].	D: Ehm, **with the effect of yoga or acupuncture on these complaints** I have no experience […].
27 SUB	I: Moi je ne connais pas euh, je, euh je ne connais pas **ce traitement-là** […].	I: I don't know eh, I, eh I don't know **that treatment** […].

In Excerpt 6, the patient has asked the doctor if there are no alternative treatments possible, such as yoga or acupuncture. In the rendition by Interpreter 2, the doctor's answer that she has "no experience with the effect of yoga or acupuncture on these complaints" (Turn 26) is simplified by means of a substitution (SUB: "I don't know that treatment", Turn 27). This renders the information less precise and makes the doctor appear less professional.

1d. False fluency

Excerpt 7. (VI-2)

18	P : Oui, effectivement, j'ai des difficultés pour euh allez uriner euh **assez souvent** et **parfois** j'ai des pertes d'urine. J'ai souvent des **infections à la vessie**.	P: Yes, indeed, I have trouble to eh go urinate eh **quite often** and **sometimes** I have loss of urine. I often have **bladder infections**.
19	I: Pardon?	I: Pardon?
20	P: Des infections à la vessie. (…) et euhm …	P: Bladder infections. (…) and ehm …
21 FF	I: Oui. Oui. Oui oui. Hm mm. Euh euh ik heb euh ik heb problemen om euh met plassen ennuh euhm ja dan euh ik heb urineverlies ennuh euh infecties, **vaginale infecties**.	I: [*French*] Yes. Yes. Yes Yes. Hm mm. [*Dutch*] Eh eh I have eh I have problems to eh to pee anduh ehm well then I eh I have loss of urine anduh infections, **vaginal infections**.

In Excerpt 7, Interpreter 2 does not seem to understand the patient's utterance "bladder infections" (Turn 18) and requests clarification (RCL, Turn 19), which she receives in the form of a clarification by the patient (CLA, Turn 20). Nevertheless, she still provides the wrong translation in Turn 21 (false fluency, FF). Moreover, some nuances are lost in the descriptions of the frequency of the symptoms ("quite often" and "sometimes"). There is also an interactional issue, that is, the interpreter mixes up languages (MIX, Turn 21), by first acknowledging the answer in French and then continuing the rendition in Dutch. Language mixing may indicate cognitive overload or stress (Section 4.3.2).

2. Omission of references to patient participation or empowerment/ substitution

Excerpt 8. (F2FI-1)

22	D: Om het nog wat duidelijker te krijgen, wil ik wat aanvullende vragen stellen over uw voorgeschiedenis en voorgaande operaties en bevallingen, om daarna wat meer **op het probleem te focussen en samen tot een oplossing te komen.**	D: To get it all still a bit clearer, I want to ask some supplementary questions about your case history and previous operations and births, to afterwards **focus a bit more on the problem and find a solution together.**
23 OM SUB	I: mais pour pouvoir procéder, j'aimerais vous poser quelques questions, pour avoir un peu plus d'information. Euh, des questions sur vos antécédents, opérations précédentes, et euh, accouchements. **Euhm, et alors, je vais essayer de focusser sur le problème même.**	I: to be able to continue, I would like to ask you some questions, to have a bit more information. Eh, questions about your case history, previous operations, and eh, births. **Ehm, and then, I will try to focus on the problem itself.**

In Excerpt 8, the principle of patient participation is not transmitted as a result of the omission (OM) of the doctor's utterance saying she hopes to "find a solution together" (Turn 22). Moreover, Interpreter 1's substitution (SUB) of the doctor's utterance "to focus a bit more on the problem" (Turn 22) with "I will try [to focus]" suggests that the doctor will find a solution (as opposed to the doctor's formulation, in which no personal pronoun is specified). Additionally, the rendition adds a layer of insecurity to the doctor's intentions by the addition of the verb "[to] try".

3. Substitution of specific medical terminology

Excerpt 9. (TI-1)

| 27 | D: [...] om u, medisch gezien, met een **vruchtbaarheidsbehandeling** kunnen helpen om zwanger te worden [...]. | D: [...] to, medically seen, be able to help you with a **fertility treatment** to get pregnant [...]. |
| 28 SUB | I: Egalement, le traitement ou la thérapie que nous on peut vous conseiller pour vous aider dans tout cela [...]. | I : Also, **the treatment or therapy that we can advise** you to help you with all this [...]. |

In Excerpt 9, the doctor specifically mentions a "fertility treatment" (Turn 27), which is substituted (SUB) by Interpreter 1 as "the treatment or therapy" (Turn 28). Although it could be argued that the patient may expect the proposal of a fertility treatment in this consultation, a professional interpreter is expected to transfer the information in a precise way to the patient.

4. Omission of expression of empathy

Excerpt 10. (TI-1)

| 100 | D: **Oké, nee, dat begrijp ik** en dat zijn allemaal mensen die in hetzelfde schuitje zitten [...] | D: **Okay, no, I understand** and they are all people who are in the same boat [...] |
| 101 OM | I: Et en fait, il s'agit des de personnes qui se trouvent, ben disons, dans le même bateau que vous [...] | I: And in fact, it's people who are, let's say, in the same boat as you [...]. |

In Excerpt 10, the patient has asked for an individual information session about IVF, since she "does not feel liking sharing her problem with other people", which she had said in the turn preceding this excerpt. The doctor shows empathy and understanding for the patient by starting her turn (Turn 100) with the acknowledgement "Okay, no, I understand", which is omitted (OM) in Interpreter 1's rendition (Turn 101).

5. Omission of expression of emotions and anxiety

Excerpt 11. (VI-1)

23	P: Et voilà en fait euh, **ça devient vraiment un cauchemar**, tous les mois j'ai mes règles qui sont hyper abondantes, et puis en … **j'ai tellement mal** que je reste alitée pendant deux jours euh, j'ai l'impression que j'ai de la fièvre, euh je je prends euh des antidouleurs et **ça passe pas** euh et j'ai envie d'en prendre une chaque heure, tellement j'ai mal. Je dors même pas la nuit, je me réveille … et euh … oui j'ai que vingt-cinq ans et je me dis **j'en ai encore je sais pas combien d'années à avoir des problèmes de règles. J'aimerais bien trouver une solution quand même. C'est handicapant presque** d'avoir cinq jours euh six jours de règles. Voilà euh, **ça m'empêche de vivre en fait.**	P: And so in fact eh, **it is really becoming a nightmare**, every month I have a period which is hyper abundant, and also in … **I have such pain** that I stay in bed during two days eh, I have the impression that I have a fever, eh I I take eh painkillers and **it doesn't go away** eh and I feel like taking one every hour, such pain I have. I don't even sleep at night, I wake up … and eh … yes I am only twenty-five years old and I tell myself **I still have I don't know how many years to have problems with my period. I would like to find a solution though. It's almost a handicap** to have five days eh six days of periods. So, eh, **it keeps me from living in fact.**
24	I: Ja, euh, ik heb hevige menstruaties euh elke maand, euhm ik blijf twee dagen in bed bijna, euhm ik heb zelfs de indruk dat ik de koorts maak, dan neem ik iets tegen de pijn, de pijnstillers heb ik soms zin om elk uur te nemen, zoveel pijn doet het. Euhm, 's nachts is het hetzelfde, ik euh, het lukt mij niet om te slapen door de pijn en de hevige menstruaties en ik, ja, ik ben aan het nadenken, ik ben 25 jaar oud, **hoe lang moet ik nog zo lijden.** Euhm, ik euh, het is ook heel hevig en het duurt vijf-zes dagen elke keer als ik het heb.	I: Yes, eh, I have heavy menstruations eh every month, ehm I stay two days in bed almost, ehm I even have the impression that I make the fever, then I take something against the pain, the painkillers I sometimes feel like taking every hour, so much it hurts. Ehm, at night it is the same, I eh, I don't manage to sleep because of the pain and the heavy menstruations and I, yes, I am thinking, I am twenty-five years old, **how long do I still have to suffer like this.** Ehm, I eh, it's also very strong and it takes five-six days every time I have it.

(Continued)

OM	
	– it is really becoming a nightmare – I have such pain – it doesn't go away – I would like to find a solution – it's almost a handicap – it keeps me from living in fact	

Excerpt 11. Continued

The omissions in Excerpt 11 all reduce the emotional character of the patient's utterances. There is compensation in the substitution of the patient's utterance "I still have I don't know how many years to have problems with my period" (Turn 23) by means of the rendition (Turn 24) "how long do I still have to suffer from this", but with six omissions altogether, the patient's strong emotions are considerably reduced in the interpreter's rendition.

6. Editorialization

Excerpt 12. (F2FI-2)

| 66 | D: Nee, maar als ik dat zo hoor dan denk ik inderdaad dat dat de pil beter geschikt voor u is. Niet alleen euhm omdat de hoeveelheid bloedverlies dan minder wordt maar ook met het achter elkaar nemen van de pil euhm hoef je niet elke maand ongesteld te zijn, dan kun je ook de ongesteldheid uitstellen en kun je ook bijvoorbeeld maar vier keer per jaar menstrueren in plaats van elke vier weken. | D: No, but when I hear this I think indeed that the Pill is fitting better for you. Not just ehm because the quantity of the blood you lose will get less then, but also by taking the pill one after the other ehm you don't need to have your period every month, you can also postpone your period and you can also for example menstruate only four times a year instead of every four weeks. |

Excerpt 12. Continued

67	I: Hmm. Si j'entends ce que … euh ce que vous me racontez, je pense que que c'est euh mieux pour vous de prendre la pilule. Euh, avec la pilule vous pouvez régler votre menstruation, c'est pas nécessaire de menstruer chaque mois. Vous pouvez menstruer quatre fois par an.	I: Hmm. If I hear what you … eh what you are telling me, I think that that it's better for you to take the pill. Eh, with the pill you can regulate your menstruation, it's not necessary to menstruate every month. You can menstruate four times a year.
68	P: Oké.	P: Okay.
69 ADD/ED	I: **C'est plus pratique.**	I: **It's more practical.**

In Excerpt 12, the doctor recommends a certain treatment to the patient and explains the advantages (Turn 66). In the rendition (Turn 69), apart from the problematic issues at the level of message content which reduce the message content in the doctor's turn, the interpreter adds her own opinion (ADD/ED, Turn 69) after the acknowledgement by the patient (Turn 68). It must be noted that this type of issue only happened during Series 2.

5.2 Interactional issues

In this category, four types of issues were annotated: overlapping speech, pauses, language mixing and reported speech.

5.2.1 Frequency of IA issues

Table 11 provides an overview of the total number of IA issues that occurred in all three series. As we saw in Section 4.3, the interactional communication level provides a context for the way information is exchanged at the main level. During this interaction between the participants, issues which inhibit smooth communication may occur, often in combination with each other – for example, a pause leading to overlapping speech.

Table 11. Frequency of interactional issues

	Interpreting method					Total	
	F2FI		TI		VI			
	abs	rel	abs	rel	abs	rel	abs	rel
Series 1	9	7.8	18	12.7	17	14.1	44	34.6
Series 2	20	20.0	19	23.8	18	14.8	57	58.6
Series 3	29	39.4	8	10.7	27	37.8	64	87.9

Note. abs = absolute frequency, rel = relative frequency

As far as the number of IA issues is concerned, no clear patterns could be distinguished across the three interpreting methods and series. In Series 1, the remote conditions seemed to have an impact, since the number of IA issues was lowest in F2FI (7.8) and higher for both RI methods (TI:12.7; VI: 14.1). However, in Series 2, only one of the RI methods (TI) showed a high number of IA issues (23.8), whereas this number was slightly less in F2FI (20) and lowest in VI (14.8). In Series 3, we see yet another pattern. The number of IA issues was lowest in TI (10.7), and the difference in numbers between F2FI (39.4) and VI (37.8) was extremely small. Interestingly, at the IA level, similar to the frequency of miscommunication at the level of ME, there is one series that shows a much higher total number of issues than the other two (Series 3). The total number of IA issues in Series 3 (87.9) was twice as high as in Series 1 (34.6) and 1.5 times as high as in Series 2 (58.6). The qualitative analyses in the next chapter will shed light on these differences.

5.2.2 Types of IA issues

Table 12 shows an overview of all the types of interactional issues observed in the nine simulations.

Table 12. Types of interactional issues

	Series 1			Series 2			Series 3		
	abs	rel	%	abs	rel	%	abs	rel	%
F2FI									
Overlapping speech	9	7.8	100	14	14.0	70.0	26	35.4	89.7
Language mixing	n.p.	n.p.	n.p.	5	5.0	25.0	n.p.	n.p.	n.p.
Reported speech	n.p.	n.p.	n.p.	1	1.0	5.0	3	4.0	10.3
Total F2FI	9	7.8	100	20	20.0	100	16	39.4	100
TI									
Overlapping speech	16	11.3	88.9	12	15.0	63.2	7	9.3	88.0
Language mixing	1	0.7	05.6	4	5.0	21.0	n.p.	n.p.	n.p.
Reported speech	1	0.7	05.6	3	3.8	15.8	1	1.4	12.0
Total TI	18	12.7	100	19	23.8	100	8	10.7	100
VI									
Overlapping speech	16	13.5	60.6	12	9.8	66.6	24	33.6	88.9
Language mixing	1	0.8	6.1	3	2.5	16.7	1	1.4	3.7
Reported speech	n.p.	n.p.	n.p.	3	2.5	16.7	2	2.8	7.4
Total VI	17	14.1	100	18	14.8	100	27	37.8	100

Note. abs = absolute frequency, rel = relative frequency, n.p. = not present

Table 12 shows that overlapping speech was clearly the dominant type of issue across all interpreting methods and series. Interestingly, within the individual series, there were few quantitative differences between the three different interpreting methods. As was the case for ME, Series 1 and 3 showed more similarities in results, for example, regarding the clear predominance of overlapping speech. In Series 2, this category also represented more than half of the IA issues, but there was a higher proportion of issues in other categories, such as language mixing (indicating underlying communication problems or cognitive overload) and reported speech (indicating increased distance between the participants), as compared to Series 1 and 3. In both Series 1 and 3, the language mixing category was only present in the TI and VI RI methods and not in F2FI. Moreover, in Series 1, there were no instances of reported speech in F2FI. In Series 3, language mixing only occurred in VI.

5.2.3 Examples of IA issues

As explained in Section 4.4.3, establishing whether annotated issues at the interactional level were problematic or not depended on their concurrence with ME issues. Non-concurring IA issues, that is, issues that occurred independently from issues in the ME and/or ET categories, were considered non-problematic, for example, in the case of overlapping speech that did not cause loss of message content. An example of non-concurring (and therefore non-problematic) IA issues is provided in Excerpt 13.[1] This excerpt was taken from the F2FI session in Series 2 (F2FI-2) and dealt with the theme heavy menstrual bleeding.

---

[1] In the transcriptions of the examples, the interactional issues are marked in bold and overlapping speech is underlined. The instances of overlapping speech of two or more persons are aligned, that is, the overlapping text is presented vertically on the same line as the text it overlaps with, preceded by an empty space. In the English gloss, the text which was spoken in a language different from the one that the interpreter was supposed to speak at that moment is preceded by an indication of that language in square brackets and in italics, e.g. [*French*]. Pauses are indicated by (), with full stops indicating the approximate duration of the pause, e.g. (.) = short pause, (…) longer pause. For more details, see Transcription key.

Excerpt 13. (F2FI-2)

73	P: Ok. (..) Et quelle sorte de pilule (.) est-ce qu'il y a plusieurs pilules hormonales, est-ce qu'il y a une pilule en particulier que (..) **que madame me conseille?**	P: Okay. (..) And what kind of pill (.) are there different hormonal pills, is there a pill in particular that (..) **that madam advises me?**
74	I: **Hm mm. Il y a plus ... euhm** er zijn heel veel ... euh er zijn een **aantal** [D: **ja**] soorten pillen, welke pil euh is er beter voor mij?	I: **Hm mm.** [*French*] **There are se ...** ehm [*Dutch*] there are a **few** [D: **yes**] kinds of pills, which pill eh is better for me?

Excerpt 13 presents two instances of overlapping speech (OS). The first one is caused by a relatively long pause by the patient (Turn 73), which is mistaken for the end of the patient's turn by Interpreter 2. The interpreter starts her rendition (Turn 74), causing overlapping speech (OS). As a result of the OS, the interpreter does not hear the end of the patient's turn, in which the patient asks (in reported speech, RS) if there is any pill "madam" advises her. This part is omitted (OM) in the rendition, as well as the adjective "hormonal" in "hormonal pill". However, no important content is lost. The omission of the utterance containing reported speech and of the word "hormonal" were considered non-problematic, since the message content was obvious from the context and, in the case of the hormonal pill, had been discussed in the turns immediately preceding Excerpt 13. The reported speech (RS, Turn 73) is repaired through the reformulation of the interpreter "which pill is better for me?". Since no problematic ME issues were involved, this instance was considered a case of non-concurrence.

Another interactional issue in the same excerpt – the second instance of overlapping speech (OS, Turn 74) – is caused by a reactive expression (RE) from the doctor ("Yes") during the interpreter's rendition. This is a non-problematic issue as well, since it causes no further miscommunication and does not require repair. A third interactional issue in Excerpt 13 concerns language mixing: the interpreter starts her rendition to the doctor in French instead of in Dutch (MIX, Turn 74). As mentioned in Section 4.3.2, this type of IA issue may indicate underlying communication problems or cognitive overload, and was therefore considered problematic. However, there was no direct relationship with issues in other categories.

5.3 Interaction management

To achieve their communicative goals, all participants are engaged in the interaction management of a conversation. They do so by following up on the turn-taking system (i.e. by taking the next turn) and by providing each other feedback on the comprehension of the information exchanged. When communication issues occur, repair strategies are needed to deal with "troubles" in the interactional dynamics (Sacks et al., 1974), for example, issues related to turn-taking, or to resolve content-related issues and return to the regular turn-taking system, in which the interpreter has the turn after each primary speaker to provide the rendition of this turn. Repair strategies range from simple repetitions to explicit requests for clarification and meta communication discussing the miscommunication. In order to avoid miscommunication and repair and to maintain the continuous progressivity of the conversation, participants can also use optimization strategies, for example, by explicitly stating their communicative purposes. Both repair and optimization strategies are fully integrated in the multimodal behaviour by the participants, which means that they involve verbal and nonverbal utterances. Together, they constitute the interaction management.

This section provides a context for the qualitative analyses in Chapter 6 by means of a quantitative overview of the frequency (Section 5.3.1) and types of repair and optimization strategies (Section 5.3.2).

5.3.1 *Frequency of RO strategies*

Table 13 provides an overview of the frequency of strategies aimed at repairing miscommunication and optimizing communication to prevent miscommunication (RO strategies).

Table 13. Frequency of repair and optimization strategies

	Interpreting method					
	F2FI		TI		VI	
	abs	rel	abs	rel	abs	rel
Series 1	14	12.2	27	19.1	44	36.6
Series 2	36	36.0	20	25.0	32	26.2
Series 3	11	14.9	20	26.7	37	51.7

Note. abs = absolute frequency, rel = relative frequency

Table 13 shows comparable numbers for Series 1 and 3 across the different interpreting methods. In both series, the lowest numbers of RO strategies were observed in F2FI (Series 1: 12.2; Series 3: 14.9) and the highest numbers in VI (36.6 and 51.7, respectively). Series 2, on the other hand, shows a different pattern. The highest number of RO strategies occurred in F2FI (36) and the lowest in TI (25). Moreover, in Series 2, the difference in the number of RO strategies between the two RI methods (TI and VI) was extremely small (TI: 25; VI: 26.2), whereas in Series 1 and 3, the differences between TI and VI were much larger (Series 1: TI: 19.1; VI: 36.6 / Series 2: TI: 26.7; VI: 51.7). These results indicate that in Series 1 and 3, more repair was needed when the RI methods were used, especially in VI, than was the case in F2FI. On the other hand, in Series 2, the remote factor had no influence on the number of RO strategies, since their number was highest in F2FI.

5.3.2 *Types of RO strategies*

Table 14 presents an overview of the types of repair and optimization strategies that were observed in the corpus of simulations.

Table 14. Overview of types of repair and optimization strategies

	Series 1			Series 2			Series 3		
	abs	rel	%	abs	rel	%	abs	rel	%
F2FI									
Request for clarif.	3	2.6	21.4	9	09.0	25.0	2	2.7	18.2
Clarif./repetition	1	0.9	7.1	11	11.0	30.6	4	5.5	36.4
Renditional formul.	1	0.9	7.1	2	2.0	05.6	n.p.	n.p.	n.p.
Meta comment	3	2.6	21.4	7	7.0	19.5	1	1.4	9.1
Correction	4	3.5	28.6	4	4.0	11.1	2	2.7	18.2
Transf. rep. speech	n.p.	n.p.	n.p.	1	1.0	02.8	1	1.4	9.1
Compensation	n.p.	n.p.	n.p.	n.p.	n.p.	n.p.	1	1.4	9.1
Change in order	2	1.7	14.3	2	2.0	5.6	n.p.	n.p.	n.p.
Total	14	12.2	100	36	36	100	11	14.9	100
TI									
Request for clarif.	6	4.2	22.2	3	3.8	15.0	4	5.3	20.0
Clarif./repetition	4	2.8	14.8	6	7.5	30.0	6	8.0	30.0
Renditional formul.	1	0.7	03.7	2	2.5	10.0	1	1.3	5.0
Meta comment	6	4.2	22.2	3	3.8	15.0	5	6.7	25.0
Correction	4	2.8	14.8	1	1.3	5.0	4	5.3	20.0
Transf. rep. speech	1	0.7	03.7	3	3.8	15.0	n.p.	n.p.	n.p.
Compensation	n.p.	n.p.	n.p.	1	1.3	5.0	n.p.	n.p.	n.p.
Change in order	5	3.7	18.5	1	1.3	5.0	n.p.	n.p.	n.p.
Total	27	19.1	100	20	25.0	100	20	26.7	100
VI									
Request for clarif.	10	8.3	22.7	5	4.1	15.6	4	5.6	10.8
Clarif./repetition	12	10.0	27.3	9	7.4	28.1	9	12.6	24.3
Renditional formul.	02	01.7	04.5	2	1.6	06.3	2	2.8	5.4
Meta comment	13	10.9	29.5	8	6.5	25.0	12	16.8	32.4
Correction	6	5.0	13.6	5	4.1	15.6	6	8.4	16.2

Table 14. Continued

	Series 1			Series 2			Series 3		
	abs	rel	%	abs	rel	%	abs	rel	%
Transf. rep. speech	n.p.	n.p.	n.p.	2	1.6	06.3	2	2.8	5.4
Compensation	1	0.8	02.3	1	0.8	03.1	1	1.4	2.7
Change in order	n.p.	n.p.	n.p.	n.p.	n.p.	n.p.	1	1.4	2.7
Total	44	36.6	100	32	26.2	100	37	51.7	100

Note. abs = absolute frequency, rel = relative frequency, n.p. = not present

From Table 14 we can deduce that the four most frequent strategies across all three interpreting methods and series were "request for clarification", "clarification/ repetition", "meta comment" and "correction". Apart from the optimization strategy "change in order", which only occurred frequently in Series 1 and therefore rather seemed to be part of the interpreting style of Interpreter 1, the occurrence of the other strategies was occasional in the sense that no specific patterns across the series or interpreting methods could be discerned.

5.4 Concurrence

To investigate the causes of miscommunication and examine relationships between the different categories of issues, an inventory was produced of concurrence, that is, the simultaneous occurrence of issues, Table 15 presents the percentage of concurring issues at the levels of ME and IA within the total number of issues at each level.

Table 15. Concurrence of issues

	Interpreting method					
	F2FI		TI		VI	
	ME issues	IA issues	ME issues	IA issues	ME issues	IA issues
Series 1	12.2%	25.0%	16.2%	22.7%	37.5%	52.4%
Series 2	4.8%	4.8%	6.0%	5.2%	4.5%	33.3%
Series 3	18.8%	10.3%	7.7%	22.2%	12.5%	10.0%

Note. ME = *message equivalence*, IA = *interaction*

Like the overviews of miscommunication, the percentages of concurrence show few similar patterns across the series and the interpreting methods. However, it is interesting to observe that in both Series 1 and 2, the percentage of concurring IA issues was extremely high in VI compared with F2FI and TI. In Series 3, on the other hand, the percentage of concurring IA issues in VI was lower than in Series 1 and 2, whereas the highest percentage of concurring IA issues in Series 3 occurred in TI.

Examples of message equivalence issues, interactional issues, concurrence and interaction management will be explored in detail in the next chapter (Chapter 6), which deals with specific challenges to the communication in RI. With a view to answering the main research questions of this work, Chapter 6 analyses specific instances of miscommunication by describing how these instances occurred and unfolded, how the participants managed the interaction and what influence technological and environmental factors had on these processes. This is done by means of representative excerpts taken from the corpus of simulations, which illustrate most prominently the relationship between message equivalence issues and interactional issues, as well as the impact of the remote conditions. These analyses will provide insights into differences in interactional dynamics in RI compared with F2FI.

CHAPTER 6

Challenges to Communication Quality

This chapter focuses on issues that touch upon several important aspects related to communication quality and which can be considered specific challenges in RI compared to F2FI. Although, as we saw in Chapter 5, many similar issues were observed with all three interpreting methods (e.g. omission, overlapping speech), their effect on the quality of the communication not only depended on the technological and environmental conditions in which the interpreted event took place, but also on how the participants collaboratively managed the interaction as well as miscommunication under the different conditions. This chapter therefore presents in-depth analyses of miscommunication and interaction management observed in the bodies of the simulations. To provide a complete picture of the interaction, for each series, a summary of the management of the opening and closing phases is provided. As explained in Section 4.4.1, these phases are of major importance for participants to establish rapport and develop a constructive relationship (Braun & Davitti, 2018; Heath, 2004/1986).

Sections 6.1–6.3 provide an overview of miscommunication and interaction management of each series that includes in-depth analyses of salient examples demonstrating the particular challenges for each interpreter and interpreting method. A detailed comparison of the three series is provided in Section 8.1. As explained in Section 4.4.3, the qualitative analysis focuses on instances of concurrence, since the occurrence of issues at several levels indicates possible communication breakdown (Bot, 2005). However, to contrast the ways in which certain issues occurred and were managed interactionally, examples from non-concurrent issues are provided as well. To aim for a more holistic approach to the analysis, comments from the participant interviews concerning specific situations are integrated (Chapter 7).

6.1 Series 1

6.1.1 Miscommunication and interaction management

As far as miscommunication at the levels of ME and IA is concerned, the quality assessment based on the annotation model showed few differences across the three interpreting methods (Tables 8 and 11). However, the increased number of IA issues and higher need for interaction management by means of RO strategies made the communication with both RI methods (TI, VI) less fluid. In the post-simulation interviews (Chapter 7), the participants also showed that they were less satisfied with how the communication unfolded in the RI sessions, especially in VI. F2FI was obviously the most successful interpreting method, generating only positive perceptions among the participants, whereas TI was generally considered less satisfactory because of the slowness of the communication and lack of visual access, as cited by the participants. VI was in general less appreciated by the participants because of the multitude of technological issues and subsequent instances of communication breakdown.

Whereas with all interpreting methods in Series 1, the percentage of non-concurring issues at the ME level was never more than half of the total number of issues, in VI (Table 15), more than half of the issues concurred at the level of interaction. This was often related to the technical limitations of the RI methods, in particular when overlapping speech occurred. Although overlapping speech led to ME issues with all three interpreting methods, the ways in which the interaction unfolded, as demonstrated by the discussion of instances of concurrence in this section, differed across the three interpreting methods. For example, in all three conditions, participants' reactive expressions during the interpreter's renditions caused overlapping speech and led to omission of the reactive expression. However, when the RI methods were used, this led to additional technical issues, especially sound quality problems. Whereas in TI, it was mostly the doctor and the patient who were bothered by the reduced sound quality, in VI, it was the interpreter who struggled most with the sound quality problems.

As a result of overlapping speech leading to sound distortions, the interpreter not only frequently had to resort to repair strategies, but was also regularly excluded from the communication when the primary participants had already understood each other and the interpreter was behind. The doctor and patient often seemed one step ahead of the interpreter. The interpreter remarked in the interview that she did not mind being behind sometimes, since according to her, mutual understanding between the doctor and the patient is the main goal of any interpreter-mediated consultation. However, the video data show that the interpreter's body language indicated stress and insecurity during these moments of miscommunication in VI (Excerpts 17 and 19).

Compared with F2FI, the number of RO strategies was higher in RI (Table 13), most obviously in VI, since with this interpreting method, the participants had to make more of an effort to ensure successful communication. The increased interaction management in the remote conditions – especially during VI – was also demonstrated by the higher number of deviations from regular turn-taking. These deviations were mostly due to repair strategies but also to the interactional behaviour by the primary participants, for example, spontaneous reactions. When the doctor did not wait for the interpreter's rendition in situations in which she had already understood the patient – especially during the short verbal examination – and took over the interpreter's turn, this caused overlapping speech and disruption of the communication flow. This type of interactional behaviour did not lead to any problematic issues in F2FI. By contrast, it had an effect on the interaction in VI, because of the sound distortion caused by overlapping speech in this interpreting method, which disrupted the communication flow. Similarly, when the doctor and patient were reacting to each other and laughing together, in VI, the sound was disturbed on the interpreter's end, causing a need for repair (Excerpts 17 and 19). The technical conditions therefore complicated interaction management in both TI and VI.

In the following, I discuss instances of the most prominent challenges to communication quality in Series 1, that is, the effect of reactive expressions and technical and environmental issues on the communication flow.

Reactive expressions

Reactive expressions in DI refer to verbally expressed reactions or "feedback responses" (Englund Dimitrova, 1997) by one of the primary participants during the interpreter's turn. They differ from direct turns in the sense that they are clearly non-floor taking. A direct turn, on the other hand, is a turn by a primary participant with the aim of taking the floor, leaving no space for the interpreter's rendition in between. The reactive expressions observed in the corpus were usually of an empathic nature (by the doctor) or an emotional one (by the patient) and occurred regularly during the interpreter's renditions during all sessions. Depending on the interactional space available (or made available by the participants), these reactions were sometimes rendered, but most of the time, they remained untranslated. This is not illogical, since it is not evident for an interpreter to include the translation of a spontaneous remark in his or her ongoing rendition, or, alternatively, find the right moment to incorporate a rendition of an expressive reaction into a subsequent rendition of a turn. Moreover, the pragmatic meaning of such expressions is often made more or less obvious through embodied communication such as mutual gaze and facial expressions. As Englund Dimitrova (1997: 158–159) argues, some feedback responses can be understood despite a lack of linguistic knowledge, and are therefore often not rendered for practical reasons:

> In general, feedback signals are most often not rendered by the interpreter, given the delayed response: reproducing such a signal may pose a problem because of the temporal and spatial relationship of the feedback to a certain utterance, which may cause confusion.

Following the criteria established in Section 4.4.3, the omission of reactive expressions by the interpreter were considered problematic in cases in which empathic and emotional responses by one primary participant were not explicitly made accessible to the other primary participant. As Baraldi and Gavioli (2007: 155) argue, a failure to translate expressions of support and appreciation between doctors and patients leads to an increased distance between them. Moreover, "the construction of reciprocal acceptance between doctors and patients", which is coordinated by means of affective support, "may be very important for the successful outcome of the interaction" (*ibid.*: 157).

In the simulations under investigation, the primary participants usually compensated for omission of reactive expressions by means of embodied communication such as mutual gaze and smiles. However, in VI, as opposed to F2FI and TI, overlapping speech often caused sound quality problems, creating a need for repair. Repair, in its turn, was more complicated in VI in the sense that it often generated a chain of additional IA issues and repair strategies. Excerpts 14–16 present instances of reactive expressions for all three methods and demonstrate differences in their impact on the interaction.

Excerpt 14, taken from Series 1, presents such an issue. The theme of this consultation was "weak pelvic floor".

Excerpt 14. (F2FI-1)

59–60 OS	I: Eh, ja, … en ja, **het hangt van de positie af** D: [*FEX; MG D-P*] **Dat is vaak zo**	I: Ehm, yes, … and yes, it **depends on the position** D: [*FEX; MG D-P*] **It is often like that**

Note. OS = overlapping speech; FEX = facial expression; MG = mutual gaze

The doctor (D) has asked the patient (P) during the oral examination whether she has pain during sexual intercourse, to which the patient answered (in the turn preceding the excerpt) that it depends on the position. During the interpreter's (I) rendition (Turn 59) of the patient's turn, the doctor utters an empathic reactive expression (Turn 60), addressing the patient directly by saying "it is often like that", while gazing and smiling at the patient at the same time. This reactive expression partly overlaps with the interpreter and is not rendered afterwards by the interpreter, leading to a loss of empathic content. Nevertheless, since the patient and the doctor engage in mutual gaze at the same moment, the patient may have been able to deduce the meaning of the doctor's message, or at least the empathic nature of the expression, from the doctor's body language, in particular the doctor's smiling face and friendly gaze at the patient. However, we cannot be sure to what extent the content of these expressions is picked up by the participants.

Excerpt 15 presents a similar situation that occurred just after the previous excerpt. This time, the patient's reaction to the interpreter's rendition of the doctor's words is lost in the rendition.

Excerpt 15. (F2FI-1)

| 61–62 OS OM | I: Ce que vous racontez est un problème fréquent chez les femmes. **Il y a beaucoup de femmes** (P: [*MG P-D ; GES P*]) <u>Ah</u> … ça me rassure) qui vivent ça | I: What you say is a frequent problem among women. **There are many women** (P: [*MG P-D; GES P*]) <u>Ah</u> … that reassures me) who go through this |

Note. OS = overlapping speech, OM = omission; MG = mutual gaze; GES = gesture

During the interpreter's rendition (Turn 61), the patient expresses a feeling of relief ("that reassures me", Turn 62), which is not explicitly rendered by the interpreter and is therefore an omission (OM). However, as was the case in the previous example, since there is a mutual gaze between the doctor and patient and the patient accompanies her words with gestures indicating relief, it could be argued again that the doctor may understand the meaning of this reactive expression through the patient's embodied communication.

The excerpts above demonstrate that all participants share responsibility for how the interaction unfolds. When a primary participant reacts in a spontaneous way that disturbs the regular turn-taking pattern, in which the interpreter take the turn after each of the primary participants, this complicates the interpreter's task of rendering complete messages. They also show that participants are often not aware of the consequences of their interactional behaviour on message transfer and therefore on the quality of the communication.

In TI, reactive expressions of emotions or empathy also led to overlapping speech several times and were usually not rendered by the interpreter, as was the case in F2FI. Similar to F2FI, the primary participants (co-present in the same room during TI) seemed to mutually understand the intention of these expressions, which was apparent from their embodied communication such as head nods, smiles and mutual gaze. The difference with F2FI was that, as opposed to the primary participants, the interpreter had no access to their embodied communication in TI, since she was in a separate location. Therefore, she could not verify whether the reactive expression was understood. It is also possible that the interpreter was not even aware of the occurrence of the reactive expressions. As a result, during these moments, the interpreter was temporarily excluded from the communication. This may have also made it difficult for the interpreter to get a sense of the interpersonal relationship between the doctor and the patient.

Excerpt 16 illustrates this issue in a consultation on "pregnancy and infertility".

Excerpt 16. (TI-1)

| 77 OS | I: Euhm, je comprends je comprends ce que vous sentez et c'est vrai, il y a beaucoup de personnes qui boivent et qui fument et qui ont des enfants. Par contre, des complications y'en a pas mal aussi mais les complications qu'on voit pas et dont on ne parle pas [*RE P: "hm mm"; MG FEX DP; NOD P*]. Euh vous m'avez demandé vous-même de l'aide pour avoir un enfant et je vous dis ce que vous pouvez faire vous-même [*NOD P*] pour faciliter **un peu le tout** [P: **Oui, pardon** [*GEST*]]. Euh, bien sûr je comprends que c'est pas facile, si vous voyez je sais pas votre sœur une voisine, ou n'importe qui le fait qui a des enfants (..). [P: **Oui**] Je comprends les frustrations. | I: Ehm, I understand I understand what you feel and it is true, there are many people who drink and smoke and who have children. On the other hand, complications there are not little either but these complications we don't see and we don't talk about them [*RE P: "hm mm"; MG FEX DP; NOD P*]. Eh you have asked me yourself for help to have a child and I tell you what you can do yourself [*NOD P*] to make **everything a little easier** [P: **Oui, pardon** [*GEST*]]. Eh, of course I understand that it is not easy, when you see I don't know your sister or a neighbour, or whoever does it who has children (..) [P: **Yes**] I understand the frustrations. |

(Continued)

Excerpt 16. Continued

78 79 OS	P: Oui pardon, je suis **un peu** (.) 　　　　　　　　[D: **Nee, dat geeft niks**] un un peu sur les nerfs. Je comprends. Bien sûr que je vais faire tout ce qu'il faut pour que ça vient … bien sûr.	P: Yes sorry, I am **a bit** (.) 　　　　　　　[D: **No, that doesn't matter**] a a bit on the edge. I understand. Of course I am going to do everything so that it comes … of course.
80 OS OM	I: Euh mijn excuses euh ja het is door alles dat ik een beetje (.) **ja** 　　　　　　　　　　[D: **ja**] reageer, maar natuurlijk ga ik alles doen.	I: Eh my apologies eh yes it is because of everything that I am reacting a bit (.) **well** 　　　　　　　[D: **yes**] but of course I will do everything.

Note. RE = *reactive expression*, MG = *mutual gaze*, FEX: *facial expression*, NOD = *head nod*, GEST = *gesture*, OS = *overlapping speech*; OM = *omission*

Just before Turn 77, the doctor has asked the patient about her alcohol and drug-use habits and explained that said habits are detrimental to the process of trying to conceive. The patient reacts to this in an extremely emotional and defensive way and seems to be frustrated about the fact that she has not conceived yet, because, as she argues, other couples who also drink and smoke – just like her and her partner –, do manage to have children. When the doctor explains to the patient that she wants to help her, but that there are things that the patient herself must also do, the patient reacts during the interpreter's rendition of the doctor's message (Turn 77), apologizing in French ("Oui, pardon"), while gazing at the telephone and avoiding eye contact with the doctor (Turn 78). This reactive expression is not translated by the interpreter, but the doctor obviously understands what the patient means, since she immediately reacts in Dutch during the patient's turn (Turn 78) by saying, "It does not matter". This reactive expression is again not translated by the interpreter (and maybe not even heard by her).[1] However, given that when the doctor says this, the doctor

---

1   Since the interpreter spoke and listened through the receiver, it is impossible to tell what she heard and did not hear.

and patient gaze at each other and smile, it appears that they somehow understand each other.

In fact, in TI-1, none of the reactive expressions that take place during the renditions, such as "yes" and "okay" (mostly expressed by the patient, e.g. Turn 77), were rendered, as was the case in F2FI-1. When the patient acknowledged her comprehension of a rendition by uttering a reactive expression, sometimes in combination with laughter, without really taking the floor (e.g. "Okay, but, well …"), the doctor proceeded with the next turn immediately. In these cases, there was no space left for the interpreter to provide a rendition, nor did the interpreter show any intention of wanting to give one, for example, by opening her mouth to start speaking. As was the case in F2FI with this type of concurrence, it is difficult to establish whether the omission of these reactive expressions was really problematic for the primary participants. The primary participants' facial expressions (smiling and engaging in mutual gaze) indicated that they had understood the utterances' intended meaning. However, as opposed to F2FI, the interpreter was at a disadvantage in TI, since without visual access, she was not able to follow the backchannelling between doctor and patient and could only guess what their relationship was like based on the auditory input she received. We also cannot make sure if she actually heard all reactive expressions.

In VI, as was the case in F2FI and TI, the majority of cases of concurrence VI involved overlapping speech. However, in VI, this was often combined with technological issues. Contrary to F2FI, where overlapping speech was quickly repaired, supported by nonverbal backchannelling (especially gaze), in VI, overlapping speech was problematic in nearly all of the cases. When two or more participants spoke at the same time, the sound tended to fall away, as a result of which repair was needed and IA and/or ME issues often occurred. Reactive expressions by the primary speakers during the interpreter's renditions were an important cause of overlapping speech. However, in VI, overlapping speech, not only in the form of speech but also laughter, coughing etc. had a detrimental effect on the sound quality in VI and led more often to miscommunication and repair than was the case in F2FI and TI. This technical limitation also made repair of miscommunication in VI difficult and often led to additional interactional issues. As a result, often, a higher number of turns was needed for repair was needed compared with F2FI and TI, as will be demonstrated by the examples below. They also show that one of the interpreters was sometimes behind in situations of repair, when she insisted on translating every turn, while the primary participants had already arrived at a mutual understanding. Again, being the person in the remote location with limited visual and auditory access to the primary participant, there was no way for the interpreter to make an estimation of this mutual understanding. In particular, when a reactive expression occurred in the form of laughter or was combined with laughter, this caused a distortion of the sound (mostly for the interpreter) and necessitated repair.

This situation is illustrated by Excerpt 17. In this VI simulation, taken from Series 1, the theme of the consultation was heavy menstrual bleeding.

Excerpt 17. (VI-1)

100/101 FF OS SQ OM META/ MIX	I: […] Euhm si jamais on donnait euh une *spirale*, une forme de stérilet sans hormones, les saignements peuvent **augmenter** [*RE* P: **Oh non, là non**; [*MG* PD *laughing*] et les douleurs aussi. Of heb ik het niet goed gehoord?	I: […] Euhm if ever we gave you euh a *spirale*, a form of IUD without hormones, the bleedings can **increase** [*RE* P: **Oh no, that no**; [*MG* PD *laughing*] and the pain too. [*Dutch*] Or didn't I hear it right?
102 RCL	D: Hoe bedoelt u?	D: What do you mean?
103 META RCL	I: U zei op het einde dat het zonder hormonen, een spiraal zonder hormonen of heb ik het niet goed gehoord?	I: You said in the end that without hormones it, an IUD without hormones or didn't I hear that right?
104 META CLA	D: Nee, dat klopt (..) [RE I: "Oké"] een spiraal zonder hormonen geeft meer bloedverlies en meer pijn.	D: No, that is right (..) [RE I: "Okay"] an IUD without hormones causes more loss of blood and more pain.

Challenges to Communication Quality   143

Excerpt 17.   Continued

105 META FF RF	I: Tout à fait, j'ai j'avais bien compris, donc une spirale ou une sorte de stérilet sans hormones aurait notamment fait plus de saignements et causerait plus de saignements et plus de douleurs abdominales.	I: Precisely, I had understood it right, so a spiral or a kind of IUD without hormones would actually have made more bleedings and would cause more bleedings and more abdominal pain.
106	P : Donc c'est le truc à éviter à tout prix, sinon je me vide, quoi.	P : So that's the thing to avoid at any price, if not I empty myself, right.
107	I: Dus dat zou ik **moeten absoluut vermijden** anders loop ik leeg (.) **van bloed.**	I: So that I would **absolutely have to avoid**, or else I empty (.) **of blood.**
108 OS	D: [DP *laughing*] **Dat** (.) dat begrijp ik. Leeglopen is niet de bedoeling. Euhm … **nu hebben we twee vormen** …	D: [DP *laughing*] **That** (.) that I understand. Emptying is not the idea. Ehm … **now we have two forms** …
109 OS META RCL	I: **Mijn excuses,** [D: **Oké**] ik heb het niet gehoord, er was een onderbreking, een storing (..) **in de communicatie.**	I: **My apologies,** [D: **Okay**] I did not hear it, there was an interruption, a disturbance (..) **in the communication.**
110 META REP	D: **Ik,** ik zei, dat begrijp ik, leeglopen is niet de bedoeling.	D: **I,** I said, I understand, emptying is not the idea.
111 REP	I: Ça, je comprends, vous vider, il faut absolument **absolument** éviter.	I: That I understand, emptying you, we must absolutely **absolutely** avoid.

Note. FF = *false fluency,* RE = *reactive expression,* MG = *mutual gaze,* OS = *overlapping speech,* SQ = *sound quality,* OM = *omission,* META = *meta comment,* RCL = *request for clarification,* REP = *repetition*

Prior to this excerpt, the doctor has discussed several treatments with the patient, who is deciding which option suits her best. The doctor explains to the patient that placing an IUD without hormones may increase bleeding. When the interpreter renders this message (Turn 100), the patient immediately utters a reactive expression by saying "Oh no, that, no!", causing overlapping speech (OS) with the interpreter, who has not finished her rendition. The patient and the doctor mutually gaze at each other and there is audible laughter from both of them. However, the overlapping speech and the mutual laughter by the doctor and patient cause a distortion of the sound on the side of the interpreter, which is not noticed on the side of the doctor and the patient. The interpreter's frowning face indicates confusion, while she expresses a meta comment concerning the communication: "Or didn't I hear it right?" (META). The doctor is obviously not aware of any sound issues and asks the interpreter for clarification (RCL) by asking "What do you mean?" (Turn 102). The interpreter clarifies (CLA) that she needs confirmation by the doctor that she was indeed talking about an IUD without hormones, as the interpreter understood (Turn 103), which the doctor confirms in Turn 104. Subsequently, in Turn 105, the interpreter repeats this information by means of a renditional formulation (RF), preceded by a meta comment (META) that confirms that she had indeed understood the message correctly. The patient answers to this, jokingly, that she has no intention of "emptying herself" (Turn 106). In the rendition of this remark in Turn 107, the interpreter leaves a short intra-turn pause before finishing her sentence, during which the doctor starts laughing and speaking, leading to overlapping speech (OS, Turn 108). The doctor's and patient's (reactive) laughter causes sound problems for the interpreter. Because of these sound quality (SQ) problems, the interpreter does not hear what the doctor has started to say in Turn 107. The interpreter interrupts the doctor's turn, overlapping the doctor's utterance (OS) with an apology (META, Turn 109) and asking for clarification (RCL). The interpreter's meta comment (META) explaining that there was a disturbance in the communication is, in its turn, overlapped by the doctor's repetition of her previous utterance in Turn 107 (OS, Turn 110). Although there is no loss of message content in the end, it is obvious that expressive reactions in the form of laughter cause technological issues, which inhibit smooth communication, since they not only require repair, but also complicate repair. Furthermore, the miscommunication leads to feelings of insecurity on the part of the interpreter, as is clear from her request for clarification, her facial expression and her constant manipulation of the mouse. In her rendition (Turn 111), the interpreter repeats the word "absolutely" (REP), as if to make sure the patient understands her. This repetition is a way of optimizing the communication, but at the same time makes the doctor's opinion on the patient's situation appear stronger than it is by introducing an emphasis that the doctor had not expressed in her original utterance.

Whereas in F2FI and TI, reactive expressions leading to a loss of information were partly compensated for by means of embodied communication between the primary participants, in this example from VI, the doctor clearly understands the patients reaction as expressed by the backchannelling between them, but many issues arise as a result of the reactive expression combined with the backchannelling. The additional interactional issues also complicate the repair.

This example shows that despite VI's potential to increase visual access, the interpreter cannot take full advantage of this because of the limitations of the image and the sound. Therefore, the interpreter faced similar disadvantages as in TI, where she could not follow the nonverbal communication between the primary participants at all. In fact, the interpreter was at even more at a disadvantage than in TI, because the videoconference technology caused additional technological issues leading to additional miscommunication, repair and altogether inefficient communication.

Environment and technology

The technical conditions in both VI and TI also led to difficulties with the intelligibility of the speakers. In VI, the interpreter chose not to wear a headset, whereas the sound quality of the laptop speaker turned out to produce a hollow sound and was therefore not ideal. In TI, the researcher had decided to use a speakerphone instead of having participants pass the telephone back and forth, since the latter option was supposed to have a negative impact on the interpreter's comfort level (Ko, 2006). Furthermore, the use of speakerphone is also recommended by Amato (2018) to allow all participants to hear everything that is being said, as they do in F2FI. However, this option did not turn out to be ideal either. Contrary to the findings by Ko (2006), the interpreter was not satisfied with the speaker mode and indicated that she would have preferred that the participants pass the phone around, so she could "follow [the doctor and patient] better". Since the volume of the speaker mode was limited, the participants had trouble hearing the interpreter, especially in combination with background noise, such as noise from the street or people talking outside in the hallway. This type of environmental factors had a stronger impact on the communication in TI than in F2FI. Since the volume of the doctor's and the patient's voices was already reduced by the speaker mode (which also caused a slight echo), noise from outside also complicated repair strategies and required more effort from the participants to understand what was being said. In these cases, the participants had to concentrate harder on understanding the interpreter. This not only came to the fore in the post-simulation interviews, but was also obvious from the participants' nonverbal communication. During moments of reduced sound quality, the primary participants avoided gazing at each other and looked only at the telephone, while they positioned themselves closer to the telephone and often frowned, as demonstrated by Excerpt 18.

Excerpt 18. (TI-1)

| 41 N | D: Ja, we weten dat euh bij koppels die in de situatie zitten waarin u euh zich op dit moment bevindt, dat dit de manier is om de kans op een zwangerschap **zo groot mogelijk** te maken. Euh, en ik kan zo meteen uitleggen wat een cyclus van ivf euh inhoudt euhm en **de belasting voor u en voor uw partner**, de kans per cyclus dat u zwanger wordt is ongeveer 25 procent. | D: Yes, we know that eh with couples who are in the situation that you eh are in at this moment, that this is the way to increase the chance of a pregnancy **to the maximum**. Eh, and I can explain to you in a short while what an IVF cycle means ehm and **the strain it puts on you and your partner,** the chance per cycle that you get pregnant is around 25 per cent. |

Excerpt 18. Continued

42 N OM SUB CO	I: Pour les couples comme vous et votre mari ou votre partenaire euh ça augmente les chances pour réussir. Euhm, moi je vais vous expliquer qu'est-ce qu'un cycle de in vitro fait, qu'est-ce que ça signifie et les chances que vous avez alors de de réussir et **c'est pour vous et pour votre partenaire** de 25 pour cent (..) **Par cycle.**	I: For couples like you and your husband or your partner eh it increases the chance of succeeding. Ehm, I am going to explain to you what an in vitro cycle does, what it means and the chances you have well to succeed and **it's for you and your partner** 25 per cent (..) **Per cycle.**
43 N OS	P: **25 pour cent de chance** de plus d'avoir un enfant?	P: **25 per cent of chance** more to have a child?
44 N COR	I: 20 … 25 per cent kans meer om zwanger te worden (.) om een kind te krijgen?	I: 20 … 25 per cent chance of getting pregnant (.) to have a child?
45 RCL	P: Ou bien dans 25 pour cent des cas je tombe enceinte?	P : Or in 25 per cent of the cases I get pregnant?
46 COR	I: Of is het dat ik in 5 … 25 per cent gevallen zwanger word?	I: Or is it that in 5 … 25 per cent of the cases I get pregnant?
47 CLA	D: Ja, dat dat laatste. Per cyclus (..) we moeten vier vrouwen behandelen om één iemand zwanger te krijgen.	D: Yes, the the latter. Per cycle (..) we have to treat four women to get one person pregnant.

Note. N = noise, OM = omission, SUB = substitution, CO = change in order, OS = overlapping speech, COR = correction, RCL = request for clarification, CLA = clarification

In this excerpt, the interpreter has trouble understanding the doctor's message, which is obvious from her facial expression (frowning) and hesitations. There are two ME issues in the rendition (Turn 42) of the doctor's turn (Turn 41), namely an omission (OM) and a substitution (SUB). Firstly, the emphasis that the treatment will increase the patient's chances (of getting pregnant) "to the maximum" is omitted, as a result of which the rendition is less reassuring than the doctor's utterance. Secondly, the substitution alters message content: Important information – that is, the burden the treatment may put on the couple – is missing, while the idea that both the patient and her husband have a chance to succeed is added in the interpreter's rendition. Apart from these ME issues, the order in which the information is given is changed in the rendition (change of order, CO), which can be a strategy of coping with cognitive overload. Towards the end of her rendition, the interpreter inserts a short intra-turn pause. As explained in Sections 3.1.2 and 4.3.2, Sacks et al. (1974) regard "pauses" as discontinuities in talk and distinguish, next to pauses, between two further kinds of discontinuities, namely "gaps" and "lapses". Whereas a pause is considered a short, intra-turn silent space by a speaker – that is, a silence in his or her turn –, gaps and lapses are inter-turn spaces which occur at transition relevance places (TRP's). A TRP is a moment in the conversation where a speaker cedes the floor to the next speaker. According to Sacks et al. (*ibid.*), the rules of conversation determine that when a participant wants to cede the floor to the next speaker, (s)he slows down his or her speaking, drops his/her intonation and hesitates or pauses, often combined with gazing at the next speaker. When an intra-turn space is mistaken for an inter-turn space by the next speaker, s(he) may produce overlapping speech. Since in the case of interpreter-mediated conversation, the next speaker is usually the interpreter, who generally takes his or her turn after each of the primary participants, the interpreter is almost always involved in the overlapping speech. This is what happens in Turn 42. The interpreter takes a pause and only then adds "per cycle" to "the chances of succeeding". Meanwhile, the patient has taken the intra-turn pause for an inter-turn pause and has already started asking for clarification (Turn 43), causing overlapping speech (OS). The interpreter renders this request (Turn 44), after which the patient immediately asks a second question (RCL, Turn 45). During the doctor's turn (Turn 42) and the interpreter's rendition (Turn 43), as well as during the requests for clarification and their renditions (Turns 44–47), there is noise (N) in the hallway, which compromises the sound quality of the speakerphone in the doctor's room. The doctor is showing quite explicitly that she has trouble hearing what is being said on the other side of the line, by leaning far forward towards the telephone. At the same time, the interpreter corrects herself twice during her rendition, which increases the confusion. This is also clear from the primary participants' facial expressions: Both the patient and the doctor are frowning.

The excerpt discussed here shows that the combination of a pause, lack of coherence in the interpreter's rendition and the overlapping speech results in repair, which is made difficult by external factors (noise in the hallway). The noise from outside compromises the already reduced sound quality caused by the telephone's speaker mode. Altogether, this combination of issues affects smooth turn-taking and thus delays the achievement of a mutual understanding.

A final example of a situation demonstrating the impact of the combination of interactional behaviour and technical issues on smooth communication in VI occurring in Series 1 is presented in Excerpt 19, taken from the consultation dealing with abundant menstrual bleeding.

Excerpt 19. (VI-1)

33 SQ	P: Perdo feminin ou Perdolan euh (.) bon euh oui (.) **Ça dépend.**	P: Perdo feminin or Perdolan eh (.) well eh yes (.) **It depends.**
34 OS RCL	I: **Euh, vous avez** dit Perdolan seulement?	I: **Eh, did you** only say Perdolan?
35 CLA	P: Perdo feminin ou Perdolan euh d'antidouleur comme ça euh (.) du euhm, comment on l'appelle encore (..) oui, pas de, oui enfin, tout ce que je trouve d'antidouleur.	P: Perdo feminin or Perdolan eh pain killers like that (.) of ehm, how are they called again (..) yes, not, yes well actually, any pain killer I find.
36 RCL	D: Is het een vorm van paracetamol?	D: Is it a kind of paracetamol?
37 OS	P: **Oui, voilà**.	P: **Yes, that's it.**
38 OS MIX RCL	I: **Oui, euh, het** ... , hebt u het begrepen?	I: **Yes eh, [*Dutch*] it** ..., did you understand?
39 OS CLA	P: C'est du paracétamol.	P: It's paracetamol.

(*Continued*)

Excerpt 19. Continued

| 40
REP
RS
RF | I: Paracetamol. Mevrouw zei Perdolan of Perdolan voor vrouwen, Perdo féminin, euhm alles wat ik kan gebruiken zei ze dan, ja, aan pijnstillers. | I: Paracetamol. Madam said Perdolan or Perdolan for women, Perdo féminin, ehm anything I can use, she said then, yes, of pain killers. |

Note. OS = overlapping speech, RCL = request for clarification, CLA = clarification, MIX = language mixing, RS = reported speech, RF = renditional formulation

In this excerpt, the doctor has asked the patient what kind of painkiller she is using. The patient tries to think of the name of the medicine and speaks hesitantly, as a result of which her voice is not clearly audible to the interpreter (SQ). When the patient pauses (PS), the interpreter overlaps (OS) with a request for clarification (RCL), inquiring about the medicine the patient uses (Turn 34). The doctor helps to solve the problem by asking the patient if it is a kind of paracetamol, which the patient acknowledges (Turn 37). Subsequently, the interpreter (Turn 40) provides a renditional formulation (RF) in reported speech (RS) to repair the overlapping speech, summarizing the previous turns, which is in fact redundant, since the doctor and patient have already arrived at mutual understanding. However, since the interpreter does not have full access to all the backchannelling between the doctor and the patient, the interpreter hardly seems aware of this and continues to translate each turn, while her nonverbal resources (her frowning, nervous smiling and constant manipulation of the mouse) point towards stress, embarrassment and insecurity. In spite of the doctor's constructive attitude, who tries to help find the right term, the communication does not run particularly smoothly or efficiently. It seems that the interpreter's insistence on translating everything (as recommended by most interpreters' codes of ethics),[2] including meta communication, actually makes the communication less efficient. As a result of the technical

---

2   For example, the Flemish code of conduct of public service interpreters encourages "transparence" by requiring interpreters "to inform all parties when clarification is asked" (<http://www.agii.be/sites/default/files/bestanden/deontologische_code_sociaal_tolken.pdf>).

Challenges to Communication Quality

equipment's negative effects on the interactional dynamics – demonstrated by the overlapping speech, request for clarification and redundant meta communication –, the potential benefits of the audiovisual channel as compared with audio-only, such as access to the participants' nonverbal communication, were in fact undermined in this example.

Besides technical limitations in the RI methods (TI and VI), another important cause of miscommunication was longer average turn duration, which was observed especially in F2FI (Section 4.2.4). Although the number of concurring issues at the ME and IA levels was lower in F2FI compared with TI and VI, the total number of observed ME issues was comparable across all three interpreting methods. A possible explanation may be found in the differences in average turn duration between F2FI and the RI methods (TI and VI). Since the average turn duration was much longer in the F2FI session (23.62 seconds) – which was almost twice as long as the average full-turn duration in TI (15.82 seconds) and in VI (14.32 seconds) – the cognitive strain on the interpreter's memory may have been greater. As has been abundantly proven in interpreting studies, by Gile (1995), among others, cognitive overload can affect the interpreter's performance. This may explain why, in spite of the smooth interaction in the F2FI session, the amount of miscommunication hardly differed across the three interpreting methods.

6.1.2 Opening and closing management

Table 16. Duration of openings and closings, Series 1 (in minutes:seconds)

	Interpreting method		
	F2FI	TI	VI
Opening	01:10	02:10	01:46
Closing	00:43	01:00	00:14

Table 16 shows a considerable difference in opening phase duration between the interpreting methods in Series 1. The longest openings occurred in TI and the shortest in F2FI. In terms of the closings, their duration in Series 1 was especially short in VI compared with TI and F2FI. The sections below describe the opening and closing management for each of the interpreting methods in detail.

F2FI-1

The consultation starts with the interpreter coming in, while the doctor and patient are already seated. The interpreter greets both and shakes hands only with the doctor, not with the patient. The interpreter sits down and first explains to the doctor in Dutch what her task is and her professional code. Subsequently, she repeats this in French for the patient, occasionally requesting the patient's acknowledgement by asking "Okay?". The patient explicitly confirms orally and by means of head nods. All three participants look at each other. After the introduction, the doctor starts the consultation. Non-problematic overlapping speech is observed during the greetings.

The consultation closes by the doctor asking the patient if she has any further questions, to which the patient answers no, adding that she is looking forward to seeing improvement in her situation. Subsequently, the doctor provides added reassurance by telling her that "everything will be all right", which is rendered by the interpreter. The closing phase ends with extensive thanking, greeting and smiling; all participants look happy and satisfied.

TI-1

The doctor and patient are together in the room. The doctor picks up the receiver and calls the interpreter. The interpreter answers the phone, after which the doctor announces she will put the telephone in speaker mode. The doctor checks asks if the interpreter can hear her, to which the interpreter replies that she can indeed hear the doctor, but that it sounds as though the doctor is far away. The doctor nods and acknowledges this information by saying "okay" and informs the interpreter that the patient is also present. The interpreter asks if it is okay for her to introduce herself

Challenges to Communication Quality 153

first, to which the doctor agrees. When the doctor is talking to the interpreter, she gazes at the device, while the patient looks at the doctor. However, when the interpreter starts her introduction in French, the patient turns her gaze to the device, whereas the doctor is looking at the patient in the beginning. When it becomes clear that the sound is quite low, the doctor also switches her gaze towards the device and unsuccessfully tries to increase the volume. The patient seems to have trouble hearing and requests the repetition of the last phrase, which she receives from the interpreter. The patient thanks the interpreter, who subsequently introduces herself to the doctor. After this introduction, during which the patient and the doctor gaze at the phone, the doctor explicitly acknowledges the interpreter's turn and starts the consultation by saying: "Fine. Then I will start now." This utterance is not rendered by the interpreter.

Towards the end of the consultation, the doctor asks the patient if she has any further questions, to which the patient responds that she knows what she has to do and that she has no further questions. The closing part ends extremely quickly. It is obvious that the doctor is eager to close the consultation, since she even overlaps with the interpreter during her rendition of the last turn. There are a few extremely short, overlapping "thank yous" and "goodbyes", during which the doctor and patient gaze and smile at each other. The interpreter hardly gets a chance to say goodbye before the doctor hangs up the phone.

VI-1

The doctor calls the interpreter via Skype video calling. After the contact has been established, the interpreter asks the doctor if she is to interpret for her, which the doctor confirms. The interpreter announces that she will introduce herself to the doctor and the patient, after which the doctor calls in the patient. They say hello and shake hands. Meanwhile, the interpreter is manipulating the screen. There is insecurity about who is supposed to take the initiative to start. The interpreter starts speaking while the patient is sitting down, but she is not audible for the doctor and patient. When the patient is seated, the doctor announces to the patient that the interpreter is present, which overlaps with the interpreter's announcement that she will first introduce herself. While the interpreter starts introducing herself, the doctor turns explicitly to the patient and gazes at her, to verify if she understands everything. The patient gazes back at the doctor and they smile at each other. The doctor manipulates the tablet during this introduction. When the interpreter has finished introducing herself, the doctor asks the interpreter if she can move her screen, because the doctor and patient cannot see the interpreter's eyes. The interpreter does so, to the satisfaction of the doctor, who reacts by saying "fantastic". The interpreter enquires if the positioning of the tablet is better that way, to which the doctor reacts positively. The interpreter does not ask the doctor and patient for any adjustments of their screen. As it turned out during the interviews, the interpreter had an extremely limited view of the doctor and the patient (Sections 7.1.1 and 7.2.1).

Of the three interpreting methods, the closing was shortest in VI. This may also have been the result of the doctor wanting to be done with the consultation. During the penultimate phase of the consultation, the communication slows down once more as a result of a sound-quality problem, which seems to stress out the doctor. She subsequently accelerates the pace of communication and quite abruptly brings the consultation to an end. Excerpt 20 illustrates this situation.

Excerpt 20. (VI-1)

125 SQ	P : D'accord, c'est bien, ça me paraît bien. Puis, oui, tant qu'on peut l'enlever, moi, ça va. (.) Voilà. Mais de toute façon, il faut bien essayer quelque chose parce que c'est tuant ce truc de règle, j'en ai marre.	P: Okay, it's fine, that looks good to me. Also, well, as long as you can remove it, for me it's okay. (.) There you go. But in any case, we must try something because it's killing me this period thing, I am fed up with it.
126 RCL	I: J'ai pas compris pas **la dernière phrase.**	I: I did not understand **the last phrase**.
127 OS META CLA/ REP	P: **J'ai dit** il faut bien essayer quelque chose parce que ça me … j'en peux plus de ce truc de règles, donc euh, voilà. Il faut essayer quelque chose.	P: **I said** that we have to do something because it's.. I am fed up with this period thing, so eh, that's it. We have to try something.

Excerpt 20.   Continued

128	I: Euhm, pff, ja dat lijkt me goed, vooral als ik weet dat het spiraaltje verwijderd kan worden zeker. Want de regels, de menstruatie da da da ben kiek beu.	I: Ehm, pff, yes, that looks good to me, especially if I know that the IUD can be removed for sure. Because these periods, this menstruation tha tha that I am fed up with.
129	D: Dat snap ik, daar gaan we wat aan doen.(.) **Tot de volgende keer.**	D: That I understand, we are going to do something about that. (.) **See you next time.**
130 OS	I: **Je ...** Je comprends. On va en faire quelque chose. A la prochaine fois.	I: **I ...** I understand. We are going to do something about it. See you next time.
131	P: Merci	P: Thank you.
132	I: Dank u.	I: Thank you.
133	D: Dankjewel.	D: Thank you.

Note. SQ = sound quality, RCL = request for clarification, OS – overlapping speech, META = meta comment, CLA/REP = clarification/repetition

The doctor and patient have just come to an agreement on the treatment that would be most appropriate for the patient. The patient's acknowledgement of this (Turn 125) is partly inaudible to the interpreter due to noise (N) in the consultation room causing reduced sound quality. The interpreter, who visibly has trouble hearing the patient (she frowns and leans forward towards the computer) requests clarification (RCL) in the following turn (Turn 126). The last part of this request is overlapped by the patient's clarification (CLA, Turn 127), repeating a part of her previous turn by using a meta comment ("I said", Turn 127). However, the patient omits the extremely emotional expression she uttered in the original turn, namely "it's killing me this period thing", referring to her medical problem. As a result, this piece of information is lost. The interpreter gives the impression of being tired by sighing and hesitating. In addition, in her rendition (Turn 128), she renders the last phrase in the local Flemish dialect when she says "I am tired of it", whereas in the rest of the consultation, she speaks in standard (Flemish) Dutch. This may point to fatigue and cognitive overload. The doctor then brings the consultation to an end quite rapidly (Turn 129), without reacting in an empathic way to the emotional content of the patient's turn. The interpreter rushes to render the last turn, causing non-problematic overlapping speech (Turn 130). After this, the patient thanks the doctor (Turn 131), which is rendered by the interpreter (Turn 132) and the doctor thanks the interpreter (Turn 133). This excerpt demonstrates some irritation on the part of the participants. Such irritations could potentially compromise a solid doctor–patient therapeutic relationship, the achievement of which is often confirmed by a satisfactory closing phase (Heath, 2004/1986).

6.2 Series 2

6.2.1 Miscommunication and interaction management

In Series 2, VI was considered the least satisfying by all three participants, despite the lower number of IA issues and RO strategies compared with F2FI and TI (Table 13). The difficult achievement of repair of miscommunication in VI and its protracted nature caused exasperation among the primary participants and thus reduced their satisfaction with this interpreting method (Section 7.1.1). This result indicates that it was not so much the number of issues and RO strategies that affected the quality of the communication, but rather how miscommunication was managed. This, combined with the higher number of ME issues in VI, had a negative effect on the success of the communication in VI.

Although similar types of ME issues were observed in all three interpreting methods, the primary participants' perceptions of the interpreter's performance seemed to depend to a large extent on their perceptions of the smoothness of the communication in general. In F2FI and TI, both the doctor and the patient were quite forgiving of the interpreter's mistakes as far as ME issues were concerned. In the interviews after F2FI and TI, the primary participants mentioned the interpreter's difficulties finding the right words, but also tried to justify these troubles (e.g. by mentioning the heavy information load and the complexity of the content) and even trivialized instances of miscommunication. On the contrary, in the interviews following VI, the primary participants showed less tolerance for ME issues and made more negative comments about the interpreter's performance. Moreover, despite the lower number of IA issues and RO strategies observed in VI, the number of negative remarks related to the quality of the communication was much higher in the VI post-simulation interview than in the same interviews following F2FI and TI. The doctor and the patient even explicitly considered the communication in VI less successful than in the other two interpreting methods. As a result, issues that were not explicitly referred to as bothersome in the interviews following F2FI and TI were negatively highlighted in the interviews following VI. For example, the doctor explicitly mentioned an instance of miscommunication in which the interpreter had not understood her correctly, whereas in the interviews after TI and F2FI, she mentioned no such examples, although comparable issues had occurred in these sessions.

The lower level of satisfaction in VI was also related to the seating arrangement. In TI, none of the participants complained about lack of visual access and no direct links were established between the lack of visual cues and the occurrence of issues at other levels. However, in VI, to allow for the interpreter's visual access to both primary participants, the doctor and the patient were each seated at a corner of the table. This particular seating arrangement turned out to be a factor that negatively affected the participants' level of satisfaction with the communication in general. As perceived by all participants, the doctor and the patient were seated too close to each another. This was considered disturbing because of the lack of distance. According to all participants, this seating arrangement was not very realistic compared to authentic settings of F2FI, in which the participants usually form a triade, in which the interpreter is seated in between the primary participants.[3]

Although most of the ME issues were non-concurrent and concurrence at the ME level was in fact lower in TI and VI than in F2FI, at the

---

3   See, for example, *Handboek basisopleiding sociaal tolken* [*Handbook basic training public service interpreting*], via <https://ec.europa.eu/education/knowledge-centre-interpretation/sites/default/files/handboeksociaaltolken_20171201_0.pdf>.

IA level, concurrence was considerably higher in VI than in F2FI and TI (Table 15). The most important explanation of the large number of issues in all three methods seems to be Interpreter 2's summarizing interpreting style. Often, the content of the primary participants' messages was wrapped up, which led to frequent omission of details, including important information about the patient's symptoms or treatment (Excerpt 7). According to the interpreter, this was a (more or less) conscious strategy. The interpreter seemed unaware of the considerable number of ME issues she produced, given that, in the retrospective interview, she explained that she deliberately omitted details or repetitions that she considered unimportant. Moreover, the interview data revealed that the interpreter was unknowing of having added her own opinion to the content by means of editorialization (Excerpt 12). According to her, she was merely clarifying matters. In the same vein, it is highly likely that the interpreter was not aware of the extent of the number of omissions and instances of false fluency either, since, during the post-simulation interviews, she considered her performance satisfactory overall, which points to a limited development of self-monitoring competency on the part of the interpreter.

Apart from the interpreter's summarizing style, the fact that she did not take any notes (which, as the interpreter explained, she deemed unnecessary for healthcare interpreting) may also account for the high number of ME issues. However, the only interpreting method in which the interpreter took some notes was TI, with no difference in results as far as the number of ME issues was concerned. Since earlier research has demonstrated that the cognitive load is even heavier in VI than in F2FI (Moser-Mercer, 2005a; Mouzourakis, 2006), it is likely that the lack of note-taking had a more serious effect on achieving message equivalence in VI. This may also partly explain the higher number of ME issues in VI (Table 8).

As the qualitative analyses of instances of miscommunication showed, Interpreter 2 had problems understanding source-text content in all three interpreting methods, though most frequently in VI. In F2FI and TI, the interpreter regularly received help from the primary participants to solve comprehension problems, mostly those related to vocabulary. However, in VI, the doctor and the patient showed less willingness to collaborate and support the interpreter in finding the right terms, which may partly explain the differences in the number of ME issues between the three interpreting methods. Moreover, during the post-simulation interview, the interpreter mentioned that while interpreting remotely via TI and VI, she found it more difficult to ask for clarification and collaborate with the other participants to find the right words. This may also explain the higher number of ME issues in VI compared with F2FI. However, following this reasoning, one would also expect the number of ME issues in TI to be higher than in F2FI, which was not the case. This result also demonstrates that the way in which miscommunication occurred and was managed had a greater effect on the perception of the quality of the communication than the actual number of issues.

In Series 2, there were only slight differences within the RI methods with regard to the use of RO strategies (TI: 25.0; VI: 26.2) compared to F2FI (36.0) (Table 13). In all three interpreting methods, clarification represented the largest group of RO strategies. This strategy was mostly aimed at repairing the interpreter's lack of comprehension of terminology or helping her find the right terms. As mentioned above, in F2FI, and TI, the participants made efforts to collaborate and help the interpreter in this respect, whereas in VI, this seemed more difficult. Although the number of repair and optimization strategies was lower in both VI and TI than in F2FI, the ways in which repair was carried out in VI, as shown by the qualitative analyses, demonstrate that the interpreter had more difficulties managing the interaction when using this interpreting method. Moreover, in VI in particular, additional issues often occurred during repair strategies, which affected smooth interaction and complicated the achievement of a mutual understanding. In the excerpts below, the issues demonstrating the most salient differences in their effect on the communication that came up in Series 2 are analysed, namely comprehension, production and repair.

Comprehension and production issues and repair

The excerpts below (Excerpts 21–24) present instances from the most salient cases of concurrence, involving comprehension and production issues, leading to hesitation on the part of the interpreter and repair. First, I will analyse two examples of these issues involving relatively smooth interaction management in F2F (Excerpt 21) and TI (Excerpt 22), which are followed by two excerpts analysing more problematic interaction management of similar issues in VI in Excerpts 23 and 24.

Excerpt 21. (F2FI-2)

10	D: Want gelukkig hebben het bloedonderzoek en de echo die we gemaakt hebben geen afwijkingen aan het licht gebracht. Dus er zijn geen afwijkingen gevonden, dus we zullen met medicijnen jullie problemen kunnen oplossen.	D: Because fortunately, the blood exam and the ultrasound we made have not shown dysfunctions. So no dysfunctions were found, so we will be able to solve your problems with medication.
11 RCL MIX	I: Euhm, on a fait l'examen de, euhm (..) l'examen de sang, un contrôle de sang et il y a pas de problèmes avec votre sang et ah ! (..) [*FEX* I ; *POS* I] et euh … l'autre … l'autre examen (…)?	I : Ehm, we have done the exam of, ehm (..) the exam of the blood, a blood test and there are no problems with your blood and ah! [*FEX* I ; *POS* I] (..) and eh … the other … the other exam (…)?
12 CLA REP	D: Echo, een echo.	D: Ultrasound, an ultrasound.
13 RCL	I: L'echo? (…) Euhm …	I: The ultrasound? (…) Ehm …
14 CLA	D: De.. de.. het onderzoek van de baarmoeder.	D: The..the..the examination of the uterus.
15 RF ADD COR	I: Hmm. On a … on a examiné votre utérus (.) et il n'y a pas de problème que, qui euh exige une opération. Alors on peut traiter ça avec les médecins … euh le médicament.	I : Hmm. We have.. we have examined your uterus (.) and there is no problem that, that eh requires an operation. So we can treat that with the medicine … eh the medication.
16	P: Donc c'est un problème exclusivement hormonal?	P: So it's an exclusively hormonal problem?
17 OM	I: Is dat een hormonale … **euhm … ?**	I: Is that a hormonal … **ehm … ?**

Excerpt 21.   Continued

18 OS	D: **Ja. Voor** sommige vrouwen euh hoort ja bij deze fase van de leeftijd, of van het leven, een heftige menstruatie. **En dan is daar niet een oorzaak** voor zoals bijvoorbeeld een vleesboom of een afwijking van de baarmoeder **maar dan is dat zo door de hormonen gestuurd** en dan kun je met medicijnen met en **zonder hormonen**, kun je dat behandelen. **Dat ga ik zo aan u uitleggen.**	D: **Yes. For** some women euh it well is part of this phase of the age, or of life, a heavy menstruation. **And then there is not a cause** like for example a myoma in the uterus or a dysfunction of the uterus, **but then it is controlled by the hormones like this** and then you can treat that with medication with **and without hormones. I am going to explain that to you immediately.**
19 OM OM OM META RCL	I: Euhm, il y beaucoup de femmes euh à votre âge ont des périodes lourdes. Et euhm alors on peut euh on peut traiter ça avec les médicaments euh médicaments hormonales [*sic*], ça on peut être, ça peut arriver euh les menstruations lourdes peuvent arriver à cause de (..) des choses irrégulières dans votre utérus, qui … euh (.) Sorry. Vleesboom? Ik ken dat niet …	I: Euhm, there are many women of your age who have heavy periods. And euhm then we can euh we can treat that with medication euh hormonal medication, that we can maybe that can happen euh the heavy menstruations can happen because of (..) of irregular things in your uterus, which … euh (…) [*Dutch*:] Sorry. Vleesboom? I don't know that …
20 CLA	D: Myoom?	D: Myoma?
21 REP	I: Ah! Myome! **D'accord.**	I: Ah! Myoma! **Okay.**
22 REP	D: **Myoom.**	D: **Myoom.**
23 REP	I: **Ah** la myome.	I: **Ah** la myome.
24 CLA	D: In Latijn "myoom". [D FEX *laugh*]	D: In Latin "myoom". [D FEX *laugh*]

Note. FEX = *facial expression,* POS = *body posture,* RCL = *request for clarification,* MIX = *language mixing,* CLA = *clarification,* RF = *renditional formulation,* ADD = *addition,* COR = *correction,* OM = *omission*

In Excerpt 21, the F2FI consultation's theme is pregnancy/infertility. The doctor helps out the interpreter with comprehension issues on two occasions. In Turn 10, the doctor discusses the results from two previous medical examinations, a blood test and an ultrasound. During her rendition (Turn 11), the interpreter makes it clear by means of nonverbal communication (hesitating, raising her eyebrows, moving her body closer to the doctor and attempting to establish eye contact with her) that she has forgotten what the doctor mentioned as the second examination. When the doctor does not respond to the interpreter's nonverbal signals, the interpreter explicitly requests clarification (RCL, "the other exam?", Turn 13), addressing the doctor, but mixing languages (MIX) by speaking French instead of the doctor's language (Dutch). Nevertheless, the doctor understands what the interpreter is trying to say and clarifies (CLA) the matter by repeating the term "ultrasound" in Dutch, which she repeats once more in the same turn (REP, Turn 12). Apparently, the interpreter is not familiar with this term and requests clarification by repeating this term in the form of a question (Turn 13). The doctor then explicitly explains in Dutch what an ultrasound is (Turn 14). The interpreter renders this information in Turn 15, together with the rest of the information from the original utterance in Turn 10, providing a renditional formulation (RF). The interpreter also corrects herself during this rendition (COR). Moreover, she adds (ADD) information by more explicitly rendering the doctor's utterance indicating that the patient's medical problem can be solved by medication ("there is no problem that requires an operation", Turn 15). The patient subsequently asks a question ("So it's an exclusively hormonal problem?", Turn 16), the first part of which is rendered by the interpreter in Turn 17, until she starts to hesitate in her translation and the doctor intervenes by already answering the question, without waiting for the rest of the rendition (Turn 18). This leads to OS and the omission of "exclusively", and, more importantly, indicates the doctor's willingness to move the interaction forward without further delay, a phenomenon that has been described in Conversation Analysis as "progressivity" (Stivers & Robinson, 2006: 386). This is expressed, for example, when one participant is trying to find the right term and the other participant suggests options or completes the sentence, thereby allowing for the progression of turn-taking (Goodwin

& Goodwin, 1986). During her interpreter's rendition of the doctor's turn, the interpreter stumbles upon a term unknown to her, "myoma", about which she asks the doctor for clarification, before rendering the rest of the content. This causes three omissions that are not repaired afterwards. The interpreter uses a meta comment to apologize in Dutch ("sorry"), thus introducing her request for clarification to the doctor. The doctor makes collaborative efforts by proposing the Latin term (CLA, Turn 20) in the form of a question, which is then repeated by the interpreter (REP, Turn 21), as well as by the doctor, confirming the term (Turn 22), and again by the interpreter (Turn 23), after which the doctor provides an additional clarification about the origins of the term (Turn 24).

The excerpt above demonstrates how the doctor strives for progressivity of the interaction and collaborates with the interpreter in order to achieve a mutual understanding, after having been requested to do so by the interpreter both implicitly and explicitly. Although there are a number of turns necessary for the clarification, the turn-taking is fast and without any obstacles. However, the three omissions by the interpreter in the turn in which she ask for clarification also show that interpreters must find the right timing when asking for a term, to prevent a loss of content.

A comparable situation was observed in TI, this time involving turn-taking between the patient and the interpreter in the consultation dealing with "weak pelvic floor", presented in Excerpt 22.

Excerpt 22. (TI-2)

| 86 RS | D: Oké. Nou ik kan een euh receptje meegeven voor euhm materiaal dat daar beter voor geschikt is want maandverband voor de menstruatie is daar eigenlijk niet voor gemaakt en dat is meestal comfortabeler, dus daar kan ik een receptje voor meegeven dat ze dat kan gaan gebruiken. | D: Okay. Well I can give you eh a prescription for ehm material that is better fitting for that because sanitary napkins for menstruation are in fact not made for that and it is mostly more comfortable, so I can give you a prescription for that so that she can start using that. |

(*Continued*)

Excerpt 22. Continued

87 SUB COR OM OS FF	I: Euh je peux vous donner euh l'ordonnance euh pour euh les pour les choses euh pour les coussinets d'incontinence qui sont meilleurs que les serviettes hygiéniques (..) [P *NOD*] euh euh alors [P: **et ... et les**] **euh vous allez** les euh recevoir ... à *l'apothèque*.	I: Eh, I can give you eh the prescription eh for eh for the things eh for the incontinence towels which are better than the sanitary napkins (..) [P *NOD*] eh eh so [P: **and ... and the**] **eh you are going to** eh receive them ... at the *apotheek*.
88 RCL	P: Mais les coussinets d'incontinence euh ...	P: But the incontinence towels eh ...
89 COR META	I: A la pharmacie, pardon.	I: At the pharmacy, pardon.
90 RCL	P: Ça ressemble à ... ça ressemble à quoi, c'est un peu comme un Pampers? (.) Parce que je me sens ... euhm.	P: Does it look like ... what does it look like, is it a bit like Pampers? (.) Because I feel ... ehm.

Note. RS = reported speech, SUB = substitution, OM = omission, FS = false start, FF = false fluency, RCL = request for clarification, COR = correction, META = meta comment

After the patient has complained about urine leakage, the doctor proposes writing a prescription for the patient for special incontinence napkins, arguing that these are better suited for the patient's problems and are more comfortable. The doctor uses reported speech (RS, Turn 86), which indicates an increased detachment between the doctor and the patient. During her rendition, the interpreter optimizes the communication by transforming the doctor's reported speech (TRS, Turn 87) into direct speech. In the same turn, when the interpreter hesitates, thereby creating an intra-turn pause, the patient interrupts by asking a question (RCL), causing overlapping speech (OS, Turn 88). However, the interpreter does not cede the turn and continues her rendition. Possibly, she has not noticed the interruption. As soon as the interpreter stops speaking, the patient resumes her question, even though the interpreter had in fact not yet finished her rendition of

Turn 86. However, at that moment, the interpreter realizes that she has produced a false fluency (FF) in Turn 87 (the term "apotheek", meaning pharmacy, does not exist in French) and corrects (COR) herself in Turn 89, accompanied by an apology (META: "pardon"). Subsequently, the patient seizes the opportunity to immediately take the floor again to ask another question (RCL, Turn 90). The ME issues in Turn 87 may be the result of the patient's multiple turns aimed at clarification during the interpreter's rendition and the interpreter's initiation of repair by means of correction. The issues consist firstly of an omission (OM: "because sanitary napkins for menstruation are in fact not made for that") and secondly of a substitution (SUB: "that you are going to receive them" instead of the doctor's utterance "I can give you a prescription for that"). These issues render the information provided by the doctor less precise and less clear.

Excerpt 22 illustrates the impact of the participants' interactional behaviour on turn-taking. When the patient did not let the interpreter finish her rendition and started to ask for clarification, it was difficult for the interpreter to catch up with the rendition of the message uttered before the request. The excerpt also shows that when the interpreter hesitates and communicates at a slow pace during her rendition, the primary participants are more likely to break in and take the floor in order to accelerate the achievement of a mutual understanding and enforce a faster communication flow, which is in line with Stivers and Robinson's (2006) observation that participants in conversations strive for progressivity. Although the repair itself is carried out relatively smoothly, without great delays, the transfer of message content is incomplete.

In VI, the same issues (production issues in the form of hesitation, comprehension issues, overlapping speech) disturbed the interaction more seriously, as illustrated by Excerpt 23.

Excerpt 23. (VI-2)

49	D: Nou ja, met de tijd dat jullie nu al bezig zijn om te proberen om zwanger te worden euhm en het feit dat we geen euh andere factoren hebben gevonden die we kunnen beïnvloeden, komt u in principe in aanmerking voor een ivf-behandeling. Weet u wat dat is?	D: Well yes, given the time that you have already been trying to get pregnant ehm and the fact that we have not found eh other factors that we can influence, you are in principle entitled to an IVF-treatment. Do you know what that is?
50 FF	I: Euhm, euh, alors euh vous vous essayez assez longtemps et euhm en général, euhm nous pensons que vous pouvez avoir le traitement FIV euhm **le traitement de fertilité intravitrale**. Euh qu'est-ce euh est-ce que vous savez ce que c'est?	I: Ehm, eh, well eh you you have been trying long enough and ehm in general, ehm we think that you can have the IVF treatment ehm **the intravitral fertility treatment**. Eh, do you know what that is?
51 RCL	P : Euh un traitement euh in utéro, c'est ça?	P: Eh an eh in utero treatment, is that it?
52 CLA FF	I: **Intéro**, oui. Oui. Vous savez ce que c'est? Euh …	I: **Intéro**, yes. Yes. Do you know what that is? Eh …
53	P: Plus ou moins.	P: More or less.
54 RCL OM	I: Euh … Is dat een euhm …	I: Eh … Is that an ehm …
55 RCL	P: (…) In **vitro?**	P: (…) In **vitro?**
56 RCL	I: **Intro** … introvitrale behandeling?	I: **Intro** … introvitral treatment?
57 CLA	D: Hmm. Ja.	D: Hmm. Yes.
58 REP META/ MIX	I: Ja dat klopt. Dat klopt. (..) **Euh oui oui c'est ça.**	I : [*Dutch*] Yes that's right. That's right. (..) [*French*] **Eh yes yes that's it.**

Excerpt 23. Continued

59 OS RS TRS	D: **En weet mevrouw wat dat** ... weet u hoe dat in zijn werk gaat?	D: **And does madame know that** ... **do you know** how that works?
60 FS	P: Euh .... **Ben**	P: Eh .... **Well**
61 OS	I: **Euh vous savez** comment on fait ça?	P: **Eh do you know** how they do that?
62 RCL	P: Euh c'est mon mari qui doit euh (..) **qui doit déposer son** ...	P: Eh it's my husband who must euh (..) **who must deposit his** ...
63 OS CLA	I: **Euh c'est votre mari qui doit faire ça hein?** [*INTONATION*]	I: [*French*] **Eh it's your husband who must do that isn't it?** [*INTONATION*]
64 RCL	P: son sperme, c'est ça? Dans dans euh allez c'est **congeler** le sperme, c'est ça?	P: his sperm, is that it? In in eh so it's **freezing** the sperm, right?
65 SUB	I: Ah dat is mijn man die moet euh zijn euh zaad euh **afleveren**?	I: Ah that is my husband who eh must eh **deliver** his eh semen?

Note. FF = *false fluency*, RCL = *request for clarification*, CLA = *clarification*, REP = *repetition*, META = *meta comment*, MIX = *language mixing*, RS = *reported speech*, TRS = *transform reported speech*

In Turn 49, the doctor proposes an IVF treatment to the patient and asks her if she knows what that means. The interpreter uses a wrong term (false fluency, FF) for IVF ("intravitral", Turn 50), as a result of which the patient requests clarification (RCL, Turn 51). The interpreter clarifies (CLA) the term directly to the patient, producing another false fluency ("intéro", Turn 52). Subsequently, the patient answers that she knows "more or less" what this is (Turn 53), which is omitted in the interpreter's rendition (Turn 54). In fact, the interpreter seems to be confused herself. Instead of rendering the patient's answer, she requests clarification (RCL) in Dutch, mixing Dutch and French in one turn (MIX: "Is that ..."). This turn is followed by another request for clarification (RCL) by the patient, who suggests the right term ("in vitro", Turn 55). This causes overlapping speech (OS) with the interpreter, who is still looking for the right term (Turn 56), but then uses the wrong one anyway (false fluency), that is, "introvitral treatment" (Turn 56). The doctor seems confused as well, and provides a clarification (CLA), albeit hesitatingly (Turn 57). Subsequently, the interpreter "renders" the doctor's clarification in Dutch (language mixing, MIX, Turn 58) by saying "that's right" twice (REP), which seems to be an acknowledgement rather than a rendition. The interpreter seems confused about whom to address. When she realizes that she has spoken Dutch with the patient, she quickly renders the answer in French within the same turn (Turn 58). However, during the pause in between the repetition in Dutch and the rendition in French, the doctor has caused overlapping speech (OS) by checking (once more) whether the patient knows what IVF entails (Turn 59). So, in fact, the doctor returns here to her original question in Turn 49, by asking if the patient knows how IVF works, which demonstrates the inefficiency of the communication. Meanwhile the distance between the doctor and patient has increased, as expressed by the use of reported speech (RS) by the doctor ("does madam know...?") in Turn 59, although during her turn, the doctor corrects herself by switching to direct speech (transform reported speech, TRP). The patient does not wait for the interpreter to render the doctor's question and wants to answer directly, causing overlapping speech (OS) with a false start (Turn 60), since at the same moment, the interpreter starts her rendition (Turn 61) of the doctor's question. After this, the patient starts her turn hesitatingly ("it is my husband, who must deposit his …", Turn 62), which can be considered a request for clarification (RCL), since it is pronounced as a question, with the intonation rising at the end of the sentence. The patient is interrupted by the interpreter (overlapping speech, OS), speaking with confusion. She renders the patient's question while addressing the patient (instead of the doctor) ("It's your husband who has to do that, isn't it?") (Turn 63). The interpreter speaks in a loud and high-pitched voice, indicating exasperation and stress. In Turn 64, the patient continues what she started to say in Turn 62, and asks now if the sperm will be frozen. At this moment, the interpreter makes hand gestures (GEST) and smiles (facial expression, FEX), indicating embarrassment for addressing the wrong participant, which led to confusion. In the interpreter's rendition in Turn 65, she produces another ME issue by substituting (SUB) the patient's question if the sperm will be "frozen" by the question if the sperm must be "delivered".

The excerpt discussed above shows that, although no direct influence from the remote conditions was observed, the interpreter clearly had trouble managing repair here. She also expressed confusion by mixing languages and addressing the wrong participant twice. Altogether, the situation and the ways in which it is managed was extremely chaotic, indicating great difficulties in collaboration and obstacles to the progressivity of the communication. Therefore, it seems that in VI, issues similar to the ones occurring in F2FI and TI, had a greater effect on the smoothness of the interaction.

Another example of this is provided in Excerpt 24, showing the disturbing effects of the interpreter's repair strategies and interactional behaviour on the communication flow in VI.

Excerpt 24. (VI-2)

82	P: Oké. **C'est obligé que mon mari vienne?** Je suis pas sûre qu'il va (…) accepter de de venir, est-ce que moi je peux pas lui expliquer, ou est-ce qu'il doit être là?	P: Okay. **Is it necessary that my husband come?** I am not sure if he is going to (…) accept to come, can't I explain to him, or does he have to be there?
83 META	I: Euhm euh, ik weet het niet of mijn man wil euh hier komen, hoe kan ik hem uitleggen dat hij moet komen? Euh sorry, ik heb vergeten te zeggen dat mevrouw dat haar man moet euh gezonde sperma leveren, hebben. Mag ik dat nog eens aan haar zeggen?	I: Ehm eh, I don't know if my husband wants eh to come here, how can I explain to him that he must come? Eh sorry, I forgot to say to madam that her husband must eh deliver, have healthy sperm. May I tell her that again?
85 META	D: Ja **hoor.**	D: Yes **sure.**

(*Continued*)

Excerpt 24. Continued

86 OS META COR ED META MIX RS META OM FF	I: **Euh,** j'ai oublié de vous dire que votre mari que votre mari si s'il prend part à ce traitement, là il doit, il ne doit pas boire et prendre des drugs, alors il doit être vraiment sain … quand il fait ça. Et si on revenons à la question de de madame, comment elle peut … euh hoe ……en als we teruggaan naar naar de … haha, sorry!	I: [*French*] **Eh,** I forgot to tell you that your husband that your husband if if he takes part in this treatment, then he must, he must not drink and take drugs, so he must be really healthy … when he does that. And if we get back to the question of madam, how she can… [*Dutch*] eh how… and if we get back to to the… haha, sorry!
87 META	D: Nee nee, ik begrijp het. **Ik euh**…	D: No no, I understand, **I eh**…
88 OS RS	I: **Ja ja ja.** Hoe kan ze uitleggen aan haar man dat hij moet hier komen?	I: **Yes yes yes.** How can she explain to her husband that he must come here?

Note. META = *meta comment,* OS = *overlapping speech,* COR = *correction,*
ED = *editorialization,* MIX = *language mixing,* RS = *reported speech,* OM = *omission,*
FF = *false fluency,* RS = *reported speech*

In this excerpt, the doctor has just explained to the patient that a healthy lifestyle is important for both partners if they want to conceive and that she would like to make a new appointment with both of them. The patient asks if it is required that her husband come. After the patient has finished her turn (Turn 82) and the interpreter has the floor to provide her rendition (Turn 83), the interpreter realizes that she has forgotten to render the patient's previous utterance in Turn 81. She asks the doctor permission to repair the omission (META, Turn 83), which the doctor grants her (META, Turn 84). However, the repair brings about several ME and IA issues. Firstly, at the ME level, the interpreter omits (OM) the question asked by the patient in Turn 82 ("Is it necessary that my husband comes?"). The interpreter also produces a false fluency (FF) in the rendition of the patient's utterance "can't I explain it to him or does he have to be here?", which is rendered as "how can I explain to him that he must come?", altering message content. In addition, the correction by the interpreter (COR) is

Challenges to Communication Quality

in fact an editorialization (ED). Whereas the doctor had said in Turn 80 that, afterwards, the patient and her partner can "talk once again about if it works out with drinking less and quitting drugs", "because that remains very important, also during that treatment", the interpreter renders this as "if he takes part in this treatment, then he must, he must not drink and take drugs", adding "so he must be really healthy … when he does that" as an editorialization (ADD/ED). Secondly, the repair is accompanied by several IA issues, that is, overlapping speech (OS), language mixing (MIX) and reported speech (RS). This makes the interpreter's rendition extremely confusing. The language mixing is accompanied by embarrassed laughter by the interpreter, who gives the impression of being insecure and confused. The doctor attempts to reassure the interpreter by saying "No, no, I understand" (META, Turn 87), addressing the interpreter directly. However, the doctor cannot continue her turn, because she is interrupted by the interpreter, who takes the turn to finish her rendition (OS, Turn 88). The reported speech (RS) by the interpreter in Turn 88 ("how can she explain to her husband") can be considered a strategy to make sure (after all the confusion) that the doctor understands that the interpreter is rendering a question by the patient and not speaking on her own account. In so doing, the interpreter optimizes the communication to prevent miscommunication. Nevertheless, this example illustrates that the interpreter clearly had trouble managing the interaction during instances of miscommunication.

6.2.2 Opening and closing management

Table 17. Duration of openings and closings, Series 2 (in minutes:seconds)

	Interpreting method		
	F2FI	TI	VI
Opening	00:08	01:20	00:23
Closing	01:05	00:19	00:12

Table 17 shows that the longest opening occurred in TI and the shortest in F2FI. The shortest closing duration was observed in VI, with TI not far behind it, whereas the closing in F2FI was much longer than in TI and VI. The sections below describe the opening and closing management for each of the interpreting methods.

F2FI-2

The opening is extremely short. The participants, including the interpreter, are already seated. The interpreter does not introduce herself by explaining her professional code. Moreover, she introduces herself by saying her name, which is unusual for a professional interpreter. The consultation starts immediately.

The closing of the session is somewhat chaotic, since in the final phase of the body, just before the closing, a certain term is misunderstood and it takes some time for this to be sorted out by the participants. Once the miscommunication is finally repaired, the doctor seems eager to end the session quickly. While the interpreter is rendering the last phrases, the doctor and patient look only at her, but as soon as the interpreter has finished her turn, the doctor and patient shift their gazes to each other, shake hands and smile. The interpreter smiles as well.

TI-2

The opening phase of the TI session does not run very smoothly. When the interpreter picks up the telephone, she does not seem to hear anything through the receiver, as shown by her body language (frowning and making gestures). The doctor asks if the interpreter can hear her and the patient, while the interpreter is gesturing (despite the fact that the primary participants cannot see her) to indicate that she cannot hear anything. Apparently, the telephone was not in speaker mode, because when the interpreter puts down the receiver and adjusts the mode, she confirms that she can hear the other participants. The doctor suggests the interpreter introduce herself, after which there is a relatively long pause. During this pause, the interpreter seems insecure about how to proceed.

Lastly, she introduces herself in Dutch to the doctor, providing her full name and stating that she works as a telephone interpreter. Subsequently, she mixes languages by asking the doctor in French "Is your patient there with you?", which is confusing for the participants, since the doctor normally does not respond when the interpreter is speaking French. The patient hesitates whether she should answer and gazes at the doctor, who makes no attempt to answer, after which the patient answers hesitatingly. The interpreter introduces herself to the patient in French as the "translator". She also informs the patient of her language combination and says that she wants to help the patient in the conversation with the doctor. Subsequently, the patient thanks the interpreter and the doctor starts the consultation. The introduction in TI (1 minute and 20 seconds) takes much longer than in F2FI (8 seconds) and VI (23 seconds). This may be the result of TI being the first session of Series 2. Additionally, the doctor explicitly asks the interpreter to introduce herself in this first session, in contrast to the following two sessions (F2FI, then VI).

During the last phase of the consultation, it is obvious from her hasty behaviour that the doctor is eager to end this. She shortly thanks the interpreter, explicitly announces that she will finish the session at that point, saying in reported speech (RS) that she will bring "madame" to reception. The doctor does not even wait for the interpreter to render this information and hangs up the phone while the interpreter is still wishing the patient "good health". The doctor seems to notice that the interpreter was still speaking only after putting down the telephone, as indicated by the doctor's facial expression, indicating regret. The closing phase in TI is extremely short, lasting only 19 seconds. This is much shorter than in F2FI (1 minute and 5 seconds), but similar to VI (12 seconds).

VI-2

The opening time in VI is longer than in F2FI and shorter than in TI. The doctor contacts the interpreter through Skype. After the interpreter has accepted the video call, she spends some time adjusting the laptop screen on her side, but does not ask for any adjustments from the primary participants in the doctor's room. The doctor does not ask the interpreter to introduce herself, as she did in the previous TI session. After the greetings and technical adjustments, the consultation starts immediately.

The closing of the VI session is extremely abrupt. After having extensively discussed the IVF treatment, the doctor swiftly ends the consultation. The doctor tells the patient that she can make a new appointment at the reception desk, which is rendered by the interpreter, who adds "thank you" to her rendition. Subsequently, the patient and the doctor both say "thank you", although it is not extremely clear who thanks whom, since first, the doctor and patient are looking at the screen, and then, the doctor gazes at the patient, who gazes back only after the doctor has already shifted her gaze back to the screen. All participants smile politely. It must be noted that VI was the last session of the three, which may also partly explain the doctor's eagerness to conclude the session.

6.3 Series 3

6.3.1 *Miscommunication and interaction management*

Although all participants were generally satisfied with all three methods, they participants voiced more negative comments on TI than on the other interpreting methods. The comments made by the doctor and patient mostly concerned the reduced sound quality, which, according to the patient, made it more difficult to concentrate on the conversation and weakened doctor–patient rapport. Moreover, all participants – including the interpreter – mentioned that the lack of visual access made the consultation seem longer and slower to all of them, compared with consultations with F2FI and VI. This perception was in line with the quantitative analysis of the video data. The average turn duration was in fact longer in TI than in F2FI and VI (Section 4.2.4). This may have been linked to the fact that the interpreter take notes during TI, whereas in the other sessions she did not make any, which made the time in between the turns longer, as the interpreter was still finishing her notes. The interpreter declared in the interview that she had the feeling she had to take more notes in TI and was stressed by the fact that the doctor and the patient could not see that, when she was silent after a turn, she was simply finishing her notes. Despite the lower number of IA issues in TI compared with F2FI and VI, the rather negative participant perceptions of TI suggests that the communication for this method was less successful than in the other methods in terms of satisfaction. Moreover, given the higher number of ME issues in TI (Table 8), possibly related to the longer average turn duration, the level of mutual understanding was lower in TI than in the other two interpreting methods.

For all three interpreting methods, most issues were non-concurrent. In fact, the number of concurring ME issues was higher in F2FI than in both of the remote conditions. Although concurrence of IA issues was higher in TI than in F2FI and VI, the low total number of issues for this method – compared with F2FI and VI – (Table 15) made the significance of these instances of concurrence negligible. Despite the reduced volume and disruptive background noises in TI, only two instances of concurrence of ME and IA issues were observed. In both cases, no direct influence of technology or environment was established. Instead, causes of miscommunication (as discussed here below) were related to the fast interpreting style in F2FI and VI, leaving very little or no space between the primary speakers' turns and her own renditions, and to the participants' interactional behaviour. The fast interpreting style influenced the primary participants' interactional behaviour, since, as a result of the increased communication pace, especially the patient, frequently reacted to a turn or rendition, causing overlapping speech, some instances of which needed repair. For example, when the patient interrupted the interpreter, the interpreter immediately started to render that interruption, neglecting what she was supposed to interpret previously to the interruption (Excerpt 25). However, despite overlapping speech and repair, only a few instances of problematic concurrences were observed and the primary participants were happy with the fast pace of the communication in F2FI and VI. The fast interpreting style in F2FI and VI was very much appreciated by the doctor and the patient, whereas in TI, they complained about the slow pace of the communication. The patient in particular felt that this slower pace increased the distance between herself and the doctor and led to distraction from the communication.

By means of a slower pace in TI, the interpreter seemed anxious to avoid IA issues such as overlapping speech. In TI, the interpreter left longer spaces between the turns and renditions than in F2FI and VI, which indeed limited the number of IA issues. However, since the average turn duration was longer, cognitive load may have also increased, which could explain the higher number of ME issues in TI (Table 8). The results of the analysis of the cases of miscommunication showed that the interpreter had trouble processing content in longer turns, since in the renditions of the two longest turns in F2FI, which were triple the average full-turn duration, multiple ME issues were observed. Moreover, during these renditions, the interpreter requested clarification because she did not remember parts of the utterances, indicating processing issues.

Although no direct impact of the technological conditions could be established in TI, the lack of visual access and the poor sound quality indirectly affected the smoothness of the communication. On the one hand, the reduced sound quality made it more difficult for the participants to concentrate on message content and weakened the doctor–patient rapport, especially in the eyes of the patient. Moreover, background noises, which were also observed in F2FI and VI but provoked no negative comments from the primary participants, were mentioned as problematic in TI, where they compromised the sound even further. On the other hand, the fast interpreting style, increased note-taking and longer turn duration in TI (which was partly a result of the note-taking) were also an indirect result from the lack of visual access and, therefore, the technological conditions.

As far as interaction management is concerned, the number of RO strategies was particularly high in VI and particularly low in F2FI (Table 13). In F2FI, almost no problematic IA issues occurred, resulting in little need for repair. For all three methods, the RO strategy with the highest percentage was clarification/repetition. However, in VI, the number of meta comments was higher, indicating that a larger portion of the communication was spent discussing the communication itself, compared with F2FI and TI. This was partly a result of the technological conditions (i.e. the loss of connectivity), which had to be resolved. Other expressions of meta communication were dedicated to clarifying medical terms and were therefore related to content, not to technological issues. Yet, neither the greater number of meta comments nor the increased clarification of the terminology in VI had negative effects on the participants' perception of the VI consultation. This shows that efficient dealing with miscommunication and/or technological issues seems more critical than the actual number of instances of miscommunication when it comes to a positive assessment of the communication quality. Moreover, the participants' collaborative efforts to repair miscommunication in all three interpreting methods showed their willingness to reach a mutual understanding.

As discussed here above, most of the instances of concurrence involved overlapping speech as a result of the interpreting style, leaving little to no time between the primary speakers' turns and the interpreter's renditions. As soon as a primary participant stopped speaking, or paused, or even when she was still speaking, the interpreter would begin her rendition. In this way, it seemed that in Series 3, it was the interpreter in particular who wanted to move the interaction forward and forced the primary participants to take short turns. Although this led to a very high number of instances of overlapping speech by means of false starts by the interpreter, the interpreter monitored the interaction closely and immediately drew back in case of overlapping speech, as a result of which the overlaps were no serious threat to smooth turn-taking. This interactional behaviour displays what CA researchers have referred to as a "preference for progressivity rather than delay" (Stivers & Robinson, 2006: 386), that is, turn-taking behaviour aimed to advance the progress of talk interaction. When overlapping speech occurs, participants tend to withdraw quickly and closely monitor the next possible occasion to resume the turn that was momentarily suspended (Oloff, 2013). In spite of the negligible effect on the interaction, the fast turn-taking style did lead to some omission of content, when the interpreter reacted too fast and interrupted the primary participants. The excerpts below demonstrate the most prominent instances of miscommunication, that is, the effects of the fast interpreting style and overlapping speech on the communication in F2FI, TI and VI.

Fast interpreting style and overlapping speech

Excerpt 25 illustrates how the fast pace of the communication led in some cases to concurrence of IA issues and ME issues in F2F.

Excerpt 25. (F2FI-3)

104
OS
	D: Hebt u op dit moment nog vragen (.) **die ik**
	    [I: **Est-ce**]
	nu al voor u kan beantwoorden?
		D: Do you have any questions at this moment (.) **which I**
		    [I:**Do**]
		can already answer for you now?

105	I: Vous avez d'autres questions que je pouvais déjà **répondre?**	I: Do you have any questions which I could already **answer?**
106 OS RS	P: **Euhm ben euh,** pfff. Une fois qu'on a décidé que … que oui, on va y aller et tout ça euh (..) que qu'est-ce qui passe? Je la rappelle euh … (.)	P: **Euhm well euh**, pfff. Once we have decided that … that yes, we go for it and all that euh (..) wha what happens? I call her again euh … (.)
107 OS	I: Dus **euh** …	I: So **euh** …
108	P: **Parce que c'est** avec elle **que je veux être**, je dois encore voir un autre docteur ou …	P: **Because it is** with her that I want to be, do I have to see another doctor or …
109 OM	I: Dus euh ja, eens dat we zouden beslist hebben van voilà, ja we gaan ervoor en euh dit en dat en ja, we doen het, hoe gaat het dan verder in zijn werk, moet ik u terugbellen, moeten we dan bij een andere dokter terecht eerst euh.	I: So euh yes, once we decided that like, yes, we go for it and euh this and that and, yes we are doing it, how does it work then, do I have to call you back, do we have to see another doctor first euh.

Note. FS = *false start*, OS = *overlapping speech*, OM = *omission*

In this part of the consultation, just before the closing phase, the doctor asks the patient if she has any further questions. While the doctor is only halfway through her turn (Turn 104), the interpreter produces overlapping speech (OS) by means of a false start of her rendition, which happened when the doctor takes a short intra-turn pause, which the interpreter takes for an inter-turn pause. However, the interpreter immediately notices that the doctor has not finished her turn and waits for the doctor before continuing her rendition (Turn 105). Subsequently, after the interpreter's rendition, the patient also reacts too quickly and overlaps (OS) with the end of the interpreter's rendition (Turn 106). The patient (Turn 106) formulates her questions hesitatingly, taking multiple micro-pauses (PS) and using reported speech (RS) in her utterances ("I call her"), referring to the doctor in the third person instead of addressing her directly in the first person (Turn 106). During one of the patient's pauses, the interpreter considers this to be the end of the patient's turn and starts her rendition, causing overlapping speech (OS, Turn 107) by means of a false start. The patient continues speaking (Turn 108) and expresses the wish, again in reported speech (RS), that she wants only "her", that is, the doctor, to treat her. This message, which is a compliment from the patient (who insists on being treated only by this doctor) that is likely to have a positive effect on the interpersonal relationship between the doctor and the patient, is omitted by the interpreter (OM, Turn 109). This may be linked to the IA issues, that is, the succession of false starts, as a result of which, the interpreter seems to have somewhat lost track of the content of the patient's message.

Although no direct link between the overlapping speech and loss of message equivalence was established, the excerpt above does illustrate that a series of instances of overlapping speech by means of false starts can have an effect on message equivalence. Throughout the consultation, the interpreter often managed to keep the primary participants' turns short by starting her renditions immediately once a primary participant stopped speaking. However, when a primary participant did not cede the turn to the interpreter and, instead, continued her turn, it seemed more difficult for the interpreter to transfer the exact and complete message content.

Of the three methods, the lowest number of ME issues was observed in VI. However, at the interactional level, the number of issues was higher than in TI and slightly lower than in F2FI. In VI, like in F2FI, the number of IA issues was nearly three times higher than in TI. The numbers in VI resembled those in F2FI, not only in terms of IA issues, but also the percentages of concurring IA issues. These were lower in both F2FI and VI than in TI. The ways in which instances of concurrence unfolded and were handled by the participants in VI were similar to those in F2FI. In VI, the interpreter's style was as fast as in F2FI and again accelerated the pace of the communication between the other participants. This led to instances of (mostly non-problematic) overlapping speech, often by means of false starts. The main difference compared with F2FI was that, although most instances of overlapping speech were non-problematic, in VI they occasionally led to sound quality problems and consequently affected message equivalence. This shows that because of the technological conditions, the interpreter's fast style was at times less efficient in VI.

An example of this is described in Excerpt 26. In this VI consultation, the patient suffered from pelvic floor issues. The excerpt is taken from a part of the oral examination.

Excerpt 26. (VI-3)

64	D: Euhm (..) Hebt u zelf al dingen gedaan die de klachten verminderen, bijvoorbeeld medicijnen geprobeerd of oefeningen van de fysiotherapeut?	D: Euhm (..) Have you tried any things yourself that could reduce the complaints, for example medication or exercises from the physiotherapist?
65 META RCL RCL/ MIX	I: Est-ce que vous avez déjà vous-même essayé quelque chose pour diminuer ces plaintes donc vous avez fait certaines exercices ou est-ce que du kinésiste ou euh (..) **excuseer** [P: kinésiste?] oe- oefeningen bij de fysiotherapeut, of ... ?	I: Have you yourself already tried anything to reduce these complaints so have you done certain exercises or have you from the *kinésiste* or euh (..) **excuse me [*Dutch*]** [P: kinésiste?] e-exercises with the physiotherapist, or ... ? [*Dutch*]

66 OS	D: Medicatie gebruikt of iets gedaan **om** ...
	[P:
	          Oui]
		D: Used medication or did something **to** ...
		[P:
		          Yes]

67 OS	I:
	          Ou euh, vous avez pris des médicaments pour ça?
		I:
		          Or euh, have you taken medication for that?

Excerpt 26. Continued

68	P: Euh non, euh j'ai fait quelques exercices euh de yoga, parce que je fais du yoga mais j'ai pas euh, ça va plus loin que (..) en fait avant je **pratiquais**	P: Euh no, euh I have done some exercises euh of yoga, because I do yoga but I have not euh, it goes further than (..) in fact before **I did yoga**
69 OS SQ	I: **Ik heb zo'n beetje** yogaoefeningen gedaan [NOD D], omdat ik dat doe hè, yoga euh maar bon niet meer dan dat want dat **is niet toereikend.**	I: **I have done some** yoga exercises [NOD D], because I do that, you know, yoga euh but okay not more than that **because it is not sufficient.**
70 OS	P: **Et pour l'instant**, je fais plus beaucoup de sports à cause des problèmes […] .	P: **And for the moment**, I don't do a lot of sports anymore because of the problems […] .

Note. META = meta comment, RCL = request for clarification, MIX = mix of languages, SQ = sound quality, OS = overlapping speech

The doctor asks the patient whether there is anything she has undertaken herself to diminish her complaints, "for example, medication or exercises from the physiotherapist" (Turn 64). During the rendition of this turn by the interpreter (Turn 65), the patient interrupts the interpreter when she uses the term "kinésiste" for physiotherapist. The patient repeats this term in the form of a question, requesting clarification (RCL). Actually, the term "kinésiste" is used in Belgian French, whereas in standard French, the term is "kinésithérapiste". However, at the moment that she was interrupted, the interpreter had not finished her turn and had not yet rendered the part of the doctor's turn mentioning medication. After the patient's interruption, the interpreter apologizes in Dutch (RCL, Turn 65) and repeats the question to the doctor. Since the interpreter expresses the apology in Dutch, it is not clear whether it is the interpreter herself who requests clarification (RCL) or if she is rendering an utterance by the patient. The doctor repeats part of the information to clarify the matter (CLA, Turn 66). The patient apparently understands the intent of the doctor's question and responds directly to her, causing non-problematic overlapping speech (OS). In fact, at that moment, all three participants overlap, since the start of the interpreter's rendition (Turn 67) also overlaps with the end of the doctor's turn and the patient's direct answer to the doctor's question (Turn 68) is overlapped (OS) by the interpreter's rendition (Turn 69). However, before the interpreter has finished her rendition, the patient continues what she began to say in Turn 68. The overlapping speech (OS) causes sound quality (SQ) problems, as a result of which the part of the interpreter's rendition where she states that yoga exercises are not sufficient anymore, is not audible to the doctor. However, none of the participants seem to be aware of this.

The Excerpt 26 shows that all participants should be more aware of the fact that in VI, overlapping speech can cause sound quality issues even if they are not always noticed by all participants. Therefore, the participants' interactional behaviour should be aimed to avoiding overlapping speech as much as possible.

As we saw in the overview in Table 13, in VI, the number of RO strategies was considerably higher (51.7) than in F2FI (14.9) and TI (26.7). The majority of the RO strategies did not involve environmental or technological (ET) issues, but were used to clarify medical terms with which neither the patient nor the interpreter were familiar. These instances were repaired similarly to those in F2FI: Sometimes repair was accompanied by IA issues, but repair was never problematic since the communication flow was hardly disturbed. Moreover, the participants made collaborative efforts to clarify certain terms in order to achieve a mutual understanding. Approximately one third of the RO strategies were dedicated to solving the unexpected connectivity problem and were, therefore, a direct result of the technological conditions. Although the repair following the connectivity problem was accomplished efficiently, the loss of connectivity did cause a disruption to the communication flow. Besides, feelings of insecurity on the part of the interpreter were observed. When the disconnection occurred, the interpreter raised her eyebrows, indicating astonishment. Subsequently, she looked around everywhere – out the window, to the door – and she touched her face and her hair, indicating stress and insecurity. All that time, the doctor and patient did not notice the problem before the end of the doctor's turn and kept on talking. Meanwhile, the interpreter was simply waiting, looking around, without intervening. Although this situation was

Challenges to Communication Quality

rather stressful for the interpreter, it does highlight that the eye contact between the doctor and the patient was extremely good and that at least they were not looking at the screen much.

Excerpt 27 illustrates this situation, which occurred towards the end of the consultation, when the doctor explained the steps to be taken for the patient's treatment. At this moment, the doctor notices that there is a technical problem.

Excerpt 27. (VI-3)

110 META	D: Het beeld **zit vast.**	D: The image **is frozen.**
111 OS META MIX	P: **Misschien ja**, ik denk dat …	P: **Maybe yes**, I think that …
112 META	D: Even kijken … Oproep beëindigd.	D: Let's see … Call ended.
	[D calls again, I picks up]	
113 META	D: Ja!	D: Ja!
	[*FEX* DPI: *smile*]	
114 META	I: Ja, excuseer.	I: Yes, excuse me.
115 META RCL	D: Ja, ik, dat dat, de verbinding … waar was u gebleven, wat had u voor het laatst gehoord van mij?	D: Yes, I, that that, the connection … where were you, what was the last you heard from me?
116 CLA	I: U sprak over een verwijsbrief.	I: You talked about a reference letter.
117 META	D: Ja (.) **Euhm**	D: Yes (.) **Euhm**
118 OS CLA	I: **Voor de** fysiotherapeut.	I: **For the** physiotherapist.

Note. META = *meta comment*, RCL = *request for clarification*, CLA = *clarification*

After the first sentence of the doctor's turn preceding this excerpt, in which the doctor explained to the patient that she will refer her to a physiotherapist, the image and sound freeze (SQ/IM). However, the doctor and patient do not notice this and the doctor's turn continues for about 20 seconds. Only after the doctor has stopped speaking, the patient and the doctor shift their gazes towards the screen, when no rendition follows. When the doctor and the patient notice the loss of connectivity by looking at the screen (which happens only 8 seconds after the doctor has stopped speaking), there is overlap (OS) in the reactions of the doctor and patient, establishing that the image is frozen (Turn 110 and 111). The doctor initiates the repair and calls the interpreter back (Turn 112 and 113), who answers (Turn 114) and apologizes (META). The doctor loses no time and skips discussing the loss of connection, immediately inquiring instead what information the interpreter managed to hear (Turn 115). After the interpreter has clarified this by saying that the doctor was referring the patient (CLA, Turn 116), the doctor does not seem to recall immediately what she had been saying before. She is helped by the interpreter, who interrupts her by clarifying "for the physiotherapist", causing non-problematic overlapping speech (OS, Turn 117). The repair is clearly a collaborative effort by the doctor and the interpreter, who quickly re-establish the communication flow together. This example demonstrates that the effect of technological issues on the communication can be mitigated when the participants make a collaborative effort to repair the issue efficiently.

6.3.2 Opening and closing management

Table 18. Duration of openings and closings, Series 3 (in minutes:seconds)

	Interpreting method		
	F2FI	TI	VI
Opening	00:37	00:43	00:40
Closing	00:14	00:12	00:13

Table 18 shows that, in fact, in Series 3, there were only slight differences between the three interpreting methods in the duration of the openings and closings.

F2FI-3

The opening is managed in a clear and relaxed manner, with ample eye contact between the participants. There are a few instances of non-problematic overlapping speech during the initial greetings. However, after these greetings, the interpreter introduces herself in French and Dutch without any hesitations or issues and the consultation then starts immediately.

The closing of the F2FI session is very short, but not rushed. The consultation ends with the doctor's proposal that the patient make another appointment with her during which she will provide more information about the treatment. The patient agrees. Afterwards, non-problematic overlapping speech occurs during the goodbyes. All participants gaze at each other and smile.

TI-3

The doctor calls the interpreter, who answers the phone saying her own name, which is unusual for a professional interpreter, who generally remain anonymous and refer to themselves as "the interpreter". Subsequently, the doctor greets the interpreter and informs her that the patient is with her. Then, the interpreter greets the doctor and asks her permission to introduce herself, which the doctor grants. During the introduction by the interpreter, the patient and doctor are not looking at each other, but either gaze down at the table or at the telephone, especially when they are being addressed by the interpreter. They are clearly concentrating on the sound of the speaker phone. The doctor pushes the volume button, without any effect. After having introduced herself in Dutch and French, the patient and doctor gaze at each other for a short moment, while the patient thanks the interpreter and the consultation starts. The introduction runs smoothly, without any instances of overlapping speech.

The closing takes place very quickly. The doctor asks if the patient has any further questions, but she does not. Subsequently, the doctor thanks the interpreter. Although the thanking and farewells partly overlap, all participants have the opportunity to say goodbye. The patient and doctor engage in mutual gaze and smile.

VI-3

The doctor contacts the interpreter through Skype. When the interpreter has accepted the video call, all participants say hello, after which the interpreter proposes, while adjusting her laptop screen, that she introduces herself. No adjustments are requested or made in the doctor's room. The interpreter first introduces herself in Dutch, then in French. When she has finished her introduction in French, the patient does not clearly acknowledge the information received. As a result, the interpreter asks the patient explicitly if she can hear her well, which the patient confirms. After that, the doctor says "fine" and starts the consultation. During this introduction, the patient and the doctor gaze at the interpreter most of the time and smile at her.

The closing is also short in VI, without being abrupt. The doctor asks the patient if she has any further questions, to which the patient immediately answers no without waiting for the interpreter's rendition. The doctor's acknowledgement of this ("okay") overlaps with the interpreter's rendition of the doctor's question, which has already been answered by the patient. The interpreter nonetheless renders the patient's answer immediately. As a result of this overlap, all participants smile. The doctor thanks the interpreter, while both she and the patient look at the screen, and all say goodbye, smiling.

CHAPTER 7

Participant Perceptions

Having looked at the qualitative descriptions of the simulations, the focus is now turned to the analysis of the participants' perceptions. As described in Section 4.4.4, after each of the simulations, I briefly interviewed the participants individually, the results of which are reported in Section 7.1. In these post-simulation interviews, all three participants (doctor, patient, interpreter) were asked to give their opinions on five aspects of the consultation, namely (1) their general impression, (2) the quality of the communication and the interpreter's performance, (3) healthcare quality, (4) seating arrangement and (5) preferences for F2FI, TI or VI. The participants were also given the opportunity to provide any additional comments. Section 7.1 is a synthesis of the participants' comments on these aspects of the consultations with the three interpreting methods. The results are presented in the same order as the analyses: F2FI, TI and VI, with an indication of the order in which the simulations took place within the series (first, second or third).

Two weeks after the simulations, the interpreter participated in a semi-structured interview in which they were was asked to comment on specific issues which came up after a first basic analysis of the video data, which I conducted after the simulations had been completed. This analysis focused on instances of miscommunication and repair and annotated comments by the interpreters in the post-simulation interviews which needed further clarification. Subsequently, a set of questions was developed for each interpreter, which formed the basis of the semi-structured interviews that were carried out with each interpreter two weeks after the simulations. The objective of these interviews was to collect more information on the background of the observed issues. This information was meant to help reconstruct the instances of miscommunication by examining, for example, to what extent decisions made by the interpreters were conscious strategies. The interviews were semi-structured and not confined to the listed questions. Depending on the interpreters' comments, some issues were expanded on more than others, or could lead to the discussion of further issues which occurred during the simulations. These interviews with the three interpreters are reported in Section 7.2. Direct citations by the participants are indicated by means of quotation marks.

7.1 Post-simulation interviews

7.1.1 Series 1

F2FI-1

All participants were very satisfied with the consultation in general. The patient was particularly enthusiastic about the smoothness of the communication and stated that the doctor seemed to be speaking through the interpreter, because "the eye contact [between doctor and patient] was so intense". The interpreter was slightly less satisfied about the eye contact, indicating that the doctor sometimes looked at her rather than at the patient while she was providing her rendition. With regard to the quality of the communication, the doctor mentioned a minor misunderstanding between her and the patient, which, according to her, would not have occurred in a consultation without language mediation by an interpreter. The doctor gave the following example to illustrate this. When the doctor announced the short verbal examination by saying that she would start asking the patient a series of questions, this was understood by the patient as an invitation to elaborate on her medical situation, which was not the doctor's intention. According to the doctor, this was the result of having an interpreter present, which delays communication and makes it less direct. In the simulations following this one, it was obvious that the doctor adapted her questioning strategy by explicitly explaining the structure of the consultation, for example, by announcing to the patient that she would now "ask short questions, one by one". This can be considered a general means of optimizing communication, independently of the RI methods, since the doctor chose to do this after this minor miscommunication during F2FI.

TI-1

The TI session was the last session in this series. Therefore, the participants often referred to the other interpreting methods by way of comparison. All three participants were generally positive about TI, although less so compared with F2FI. Negative aspects that were mentioned (mainly by the doctor and the patient) concerned the perceived slowness of the communication and the increased social distance between the primary participants.

The doctor mentioned the lack of visual cues in TI as a major disadvantage. According to her, this was the main factor slowing down the communication, since during the interpreter's pauses, she had no clue whether the interpreter had finished speaking or not. As she said, this was different in VI, because the webcam allowed the participants to see what the interpreter was doing, for example, taking notes. This lack of visual access created greater distance between the participants and rendered the communication unnatural, according to the doctor.

The patient also mentioned the issue of increased distance and added that she sometimes had forgotten what had been said at the beginning of a given turn because of the delayed communication. In fact, the patient provided the highest number of negative comments on TI of all three participants, and also mentioned the impossibility of expressing spontaneous reactions and the detachment from the communication as a result of the use of a "machine". She was bothered by the fact that she and the doctor were gazing at the telephone instead of at each other. Yet, since there were fewer "hitches" in the communication in TI, the patient did evaluate this interpreting method more positive than VI. According to her, during TI, she at least did not feel that her attention was "distracted by seeing the image of the interpreter" (as was the case in VI) and was able to "focus better on the words of the interpreter".

The interpreter was much more positive about the TI session than the doctor and patient had been. Although she also mentioned the lack of visual access to the embodied communication, which, for example, made it difficult for her to "assess emotional reactions", the interpreter claimed that she felt more in control of the interaction in TI than in F2FI and VI. She explained that, since the communication seemed slower in TI and there was little room for spontaneous reactions, she felt more in charge of the communication management. By speaking in a slow and deliberate manner, she felt better able to steer the communication in this interpreting method compared with F2FI and VI, because in this way, she forced the participants to wait for her to finish. The interpreter also mentioned the issue of detachment from the other participants, in line with what the patient had cited. However, contrary to the patient, the interpreter perceived this detachment rather as an advantage of TI compared with VI and F2FI. According to the interpreter, in general, interlocutors are "less likely to engage in side-talk with her in TI", which, in the interpreter's words, allows her to be "more neutral".

Whereas the patient and doctor saw no impact on the quality of care in TI, the interpreter mentioned that she had the impression that "the patient may have had additional questions, which she did not ask in TI but possibly might have asked in F2FI", since the conversation "ran more smoothly" in F2FI.

As far as technology was concerned, none of the participants explicitly mentioned the reduced sound quality in TI as a negative aspect. This is surprising, given the findings of the objective assessment, which revealed a number of IA issues as a result of sound quality. However, the lack of visual access in TI and the lack of eye contact between the doctor and the patient during TI (mentioned by the patient in particular) were considered obstacles to the communication.

VI-1

The VI session in Series 1 generated more varying perceptions among the participants than F2FI and TI. Although all the participants claimed that their general satisfaction with the consultation was "sufficient", the remarks by the patient and the interpreter were mostly negative. The only participant who was moderately positive in general was the doctor, who appeared to be less bothered by the regularly occurring communication breakdowns. The doctor was also particularly favourable to the advantages of VI with respect to cost-efficiency, and said she would be happy to introduce VI in her practice to save the time and cost associated with hiring a face-to-face interpreter. The doctor also remarked that, as opposed to TI, pauses and silences were not a problem in VI, because she could tell from the interpreter's body language when she had finished her renditions. The doctor therefore largely preferred the audiovisual channel to audio-only. She also thought that the audiovisual channel better accommodates "the way we communicate nowadays" and that the quality of care was not affected by the communication channel. Contrary to the patient and the interpreter, the doctor felt that, despite some "hitches" in the communication, after which the communication went "every which way", the interaction between the participants was good. Despite the participants' general impression of VI being "sufficient", the comments by the patient and the interpreter were mostly negative. The interpreter felt that the quality of the communication and healthcare was "reduced" with this interpreting method. According to the interpreter, because of the bad sound and image quality, "some of the content got lost" and she had the impression that she had to resort to summarizing the utterances. The interpreter also mentioned that, in her opinion, VI definitely does have advantages, such as "more neutrality" compared with F2FI. Moreover, she felt the success of VI also "depends on the subject of the consultation", giving the example that bad news or intimate subjects "makes some consultations more appropriate to VI than others". Furthermore, both patient and interpreter complained about the technical conditions in VI, for example, the reduced sound quality and the seating arrangement. Figure 4 shows the views of two of the cameras (on the left, a centre view of the doctor and patient, and on the right, a view of the interpreter) in the way they were synchronized in ELAN for annotation.

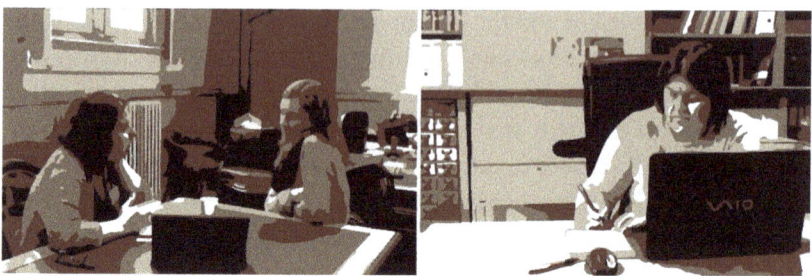

Figure 4. Seating arrangement in VI-1.

The interpreter mentioned that she was bothered by the lack of a full view of the doctor and patient on her laptop. This is somewhat contradictory to the doctor's comments, who claimed that she had checked that both she and the patient were visible on the picture-in-picture on their tablet screen. Whereas during the introductory phase of the consultation, the doctor asked the interpreter to move her screen to be able to have a better view, the interpreter claimed in the interview that there was no space for her to do the same, as she "had to put all her energy in the interpreting". However, the video data show that the pace of the introduction was not particularly hurried. Therefore, the fact that the interpreter did not ask for technical adjustments may rather be due to a lack of experience with VI and of a clear protocol for VI sessions than a lack of opportunity to request these adjustments. The interpreter also remarked that, in her opinion, VI could be a successful means of communication, but that "the technical standards of VI", meaning the VC software used in the simulations, are "not yet sufficient to support smooth communication".

The patient's objections to the VI method were in line with the interpreter's. In addition, the patient mentioned experiencing an even greater distance between her and the doctor in VI than in TI, probably as a result of frequent communication breakdown. According to the patient, since too much attention had to be attributed to the communication medium, she and the doctor did not manage "to make a connection". As a result, the patient perceived the quality of the provided healthcare as "less good" and felt "less reassured and understood" by the doctor than in F2FI

Participant Perceptions 193

and TI. According to the patient, this was true for both TI and VI, though she felt the interpreter was more present (in a negative sense) during VI than during TI. Since communication breakdown was most frequent in VI, more repair was needed than in F2FI and TI. This drew more attention to the mediated character of the communication (as opposed to direct, communication that is not mediated by an interpreter) and increased the presence and visibility of the interpreter, according to the patient.

7.1.2 Series 2

F2FI-2

Whereas the interpreter was "very satisfied" with the consultation in general, both the doctor and the patient were merely "rather positive".[1] The doctor expressed doubts about the interpreter's "translations", and mentioned, for example, a shift in meaning when the possibility of thrombosis was discussed. The doctor also noticed that the interpreter did not take notes, "despite the heavy information load", as the doctor argued. In the same vein, the patient mentioned that, "especially considering the complexity of the subject", the interpreter did her job "very well". None of the participants felt that there were moments when the communication flow was disturbed. Both primary participants were satisfied with the quality of care.

Although the interpreter claimed to be very satisfied with the consultation in general, as well as with her own performance, she blamed herself for not finding the right words from time to time. However, she said that she had been "happy to receive help" from the other participants in these situations. Interestingly, the interpreter also mentioned that, during F2FI, she found it easier to ask questions than during the RI sessions. This may also explain the higher number of RO strategies in F2FI compared with

---

1   It must be noted that the simulations of Series 2 and 3 took place on the same day. As a result, in the interviews, the participants tended to make comparisons between Interpreters 2 and 3, but made no comparison with Interpreter 1, since Series 1 had taken place a few months before.

TI and VI (Table 13), particularly the higher number of requests for clarification (Table 14).

All three participants preferred F2FI to TI and VI, citing reasons such as F2FI being "more human" and allowing for visual access. The patient also mentioned eye contact as an important advantage of F2FI, whereas the interpreter spoke of the "personal and friendly" nature of live communication in F2FI. She also mentioned the benefits of full access to facial expressions, which, according to the interpreter, "helped to interpret how a message was intended".

TI-2

All three participants were "rather positive" about TI. The doctor mentioned that the beginning was difficult and that it took some time for the interpreter to "warm up". According to the doctor, the interpreter often had to search for the right terms, which "slowed down the communication". However, the doctor also mentioned that this did not bother her much. The patient also experienced the communication as "more difficult" at the beginning of the consultation. Moreover, she had the impression that the interpreter was "extremely stressed" and did not look "at ease", as a result of which "the communication was not always clear" and some of the terms were wrong, according to the patient. The patient said that, as a result of the wrong term, she was not exactly sure about what she had to do or whom to turn to. She did emphasize that this instance of uncertainty was the only moment of misunderstanding. The interpreter herself also admitted that she often had to search for words, which she blamed on the fact that French is her second working language, which she uses less often than her other working language. Although they were not specifically asked about this, both the interpreter and the patient complimented the doctor's communication skills, which they both described as "excellent".

Concerning technology, all participants mentioned that they had not been bothered by the lack of visual access. Although the interpreter stated that she preferred F2FI to TI, she mentioned that, in her daily work, she practices TI much more frequently than F2FI. Consequently, she is very much used to this interpreting method and commented that the lack of visual access was "no issue" for her. The participants did voice a number of negative comments about technical aspects, in particular the speakerphone's sound quality. The doctor said that the sound was "tinny" and sometimes "creaky". She was able to hear the interpreter, but she felt as if she had to make "an extra effort" to understand what was being said. The interpreter was also bothered by the sound, mainly when the patient spoke, because, according to the interpreter, the patient's voice quality did not carry as well as the doctor's. The patient found the sound quality of the telephone "limited". To her, the interpreter sounded far away, "as if she was in Africa or something". Also with regard to technological issues, the patient remarked that she found it strange to "talk to a machine", which made the communication "less human" to her. Although she claimed that she felt at ease during the TI session, she found it difficult that she was not able "to react more spontaneously".

VI-2

In VI, the levels of satisfaction with the consultation in general varied among participants. Whereas the interpreter was "satisfied", the doctor considered the consultation "okay, but much less good than the other two sessions". The patient claimed to be "averagely satisfied, neither positive, nor negative". During these interviews, many more negative remarks were made than during the interviews after F2FI and TI. The doctor specifically mentioned several shifts in meaning that she had observed herself, for example, when she discussed the chance of conceiving, which was "not simply 15%, but 15% every month". She also remarked that the interpreter corrected herself regularly, which made the interpreter less reliable in the eyes of the doctor. Furthermore, the doctor complained about the confusion caused by the interpreter's language mixing, sometimes addressing the doctor in French or the patient in Dutch. This issue was also mentioned by the patient, who stated that sometimes she was "not sure whose turn it was to speak". Like the doctor, the patient had doubts about the accuracy of the renditions. The patient also provided a few examples of this, one of them being the interpreter saying "manière de vie" [manner of living] instead of "style de vie" [lifestyle]. The patient criticized this rendition, since, according to her, it made the doctor's words sound "like an attack". According to the patient, the doctor's communication was gentle and soft, so she had trouble imagining the doctor using this term. The patient also felt that the doctor had probably not understood everything that the patient had said during the consultation, because of "all the miscomprehension". The fact that the patient thought the interpreter "did a good job" is therefore almost contradictory. In addition, despite the large number of negative remarks from both the patient and the doctor, the primary participants did find the quality of care to be "satisfactory". As was the case in the interviews after F2FI and TI, the interpreter mentioned as a negative point that she had sometimes had to search for the right terms, but also said that, generally speaking, "everyone understood everyone".

Contrary to what was the case in F2FI and TI, both doctor and patient mentioned that they found it difficult to "connect" with each other in VI. The doctor said that this interpreting method made it difficult "to get in touch" with the patient compared with the other two methods, mostly because of how they were seated, but also because of the subject of the VI consultation, which was the most difficult of all three consultations, according to the doctor. "Giving lifestyle advice to people who are not open to it is never an easy task", the doctor argued. Whereas in the other two scenarios a treatment was discussed or medication prescribed, "in this scenario, the patient goes home with something she does not like and which is difficult, that is, changing her lifestyle".

While in F2FI and TI, the seating arrangement was considered "satisfactory" and no explicit remarks were made on the subject, during VI, the constellation – with the doctor and patient being rather close to one another in order to have both of their faces on the screen – was very much criticized by all three participants. Figure 5 illustrates the seating arrangement in VI. It shows the doctor and the patient on the left, the interpreter in the middle and the view from the interpreter's screen on the right.

Participant Perceptions

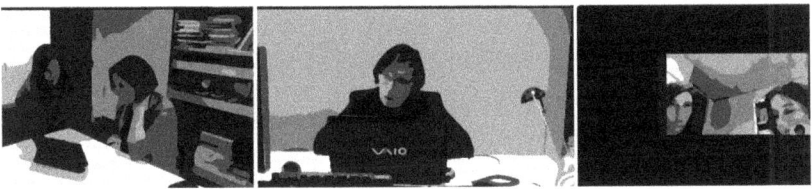

Figure 5. Seating arrangement in VI-2.

For the doctor, the lack of distance between her and the patient was an extremely negative point, which she repeated several times. The seating arrangement made it more difficult for her to create some distance when the patient behaved in a "rather unpleasant and defensive way". As the doctor commented, "in a normal, face-to-face consultation, the doctor and patient are opposite each other", which makes it easier "to be more authoritative". According to the doctor, this professional distance is needed "to keep it business-like". The interpreter said that the view of the doctor and patient, next to each other instead of opposite each other, was unnatural and "made them look like friends".

As far as the technological conditions were concerned, none of the participants mentioned any potential negative effects of technology on the communication, apart from a few moments of poor sound quality. According to the doctor, these instances "did not influence comprehensibility". As was the case in TI, the interpreter mentioned that she was sometimes bothered by the patient's poor audibility. The interpreter mentioned that an advantage of VI was having visual access to the primary speakers (as opposed to TI), which helped her to "interpret facial expressions". When questioned about her preference, the doctor expressed her preference for VI over TI mentioning visual access, as long as the quality of the video technology was "acceptable". Interestingly enough, the doctor seemed more inclined to accept certain negative aspects of VI, such as the delay in the transfer of sound and image and potential concomitant repair. According to her, there must be "a good balance between the costs and quality of the communication, but if the costs are significantly lower when using a video interpreter compared to a face-to-face one, a slightly poorer quality may be acceptable".

7.1.3 Series 3

F2FI-3

All three participants' overall impression of the F2FI consultation was positive in Series 3. The doctor commented that "the interaction with the interpreter ran very smoothly" and that "the interpreter was dividing her attention and eye contact very well between me and the patient, and she was really following the patient's emotions". When asked about possible negative aspects, neither the doctor or the patient voiced any negative comments, whereas the interpreter referred to her own performance and mentioned the fact that she had to ask for clarification once or twice. According to the interpreter, the terminology in the F2FI consultation was "complicated", although during the same interview, she also called it "a normal assignment" and remarked that all three consultation themes were "equally complicated" as far as terminology was concerned. Later, the interpreter again contradicted herself in the interview after TI and in the in-depth interview two weeks after the simulation when she stated that the content of the TI consultation was more complicated and that she had the impression the doctor was speaking faster in the TI consultation. This suggests that the lack of visual access in TI affected the interpreter's perception of the quality of the communication.

The participants were also positive about the quality of the communication. All found that a mutual understanding was achieved. Both the patient and the interpreter voiced that the clarification of the term "prescription" was the only moment during the F2FI consultation that the communication flow was interrupted. However, they also said that the issue was solved quickly. When asked if they found the quality of care to be sufficient and whether there was enough room for the patient to ask questions, all participants confirmed this. The doctor, the patient and the interpreter all agreed that the triadic constellation was appropriate. When asked about their preferences, the doctor remarked that she had a "very slight preference for F2FI", but added that "it depends on the interpreter". She explained: "If the interpreter is less good, there is a greater need for F2FI, because you need more nonverbal communication to understand."

She also mentioned that, in real life, the decision to use VI instead of F2FI would depend on the subject of the consultation, since, according to the doctor, "for bad news consultations, VI is obviously not appropriate". The patient expressed similar remarks and commented that "with this interpreter", there were hardly any differences between F2FI and VI. Therefore, between these two interpreting methods, the patient had no preference for one or the other. As far as the interpreter was concerned, she considered that each of the three interpreting methods had "its own specific advantages". The interpreter also remarked that she did not notice many differences between F2FI and VI.

TI-3

Although all participants claimed to have an overall positive impression of the TI consultation, more negative remarks were made about TI than about F2FI and VI, especially by the doctor and the patient. These remarks were mainly related to the sound quality of the speakerphone. The doctor remarked that her overall impression of the TI session was "only good, because the interpreter was so careful and I heard her following [us] closely while she was taking notes". Negative comments by the interpreter were once again related to her own performance, for example, her use of a wrong term. However, the interpreter stressed that this negative comment was not related to the fact that the interpreting took place via telephone. Interestingly, all three participants claimed to be satisfied with the communication and the interpreter's performance, but all mentioned the same terminological issue, which made the communication momentarily run less smooth in their eyes. However, according to the doctor, the issue was "solved by itself".

The quality of care and seating arrangement were deemed sufficient by all participants. As far the technological conditions were concerned, as mentioned before, the patient and the doctor were bothered by the reduced volume and the noise from the construction work outside the building. The interpreter mentioned the lack of visual access as a negative factor in TI. She explained that when she practices TI in her daily professional life, she has the habit of taking more notes than in F2FI and that she finds it stressful in TI in general that the other participants cannot see that, after they have stopped talking, the interpreter still has to finish her notes. The doctor claimed not to be bothered "so much" by the lack of visual access, but did remark that the silences in between the turns (when the interpreter was finishing her notes) could have seemed less long had she been able to see the interpreter. "You don't know if the silences come from writing, thinking or her waiting to be sure we had finished talking." In terms of technology, the patient linked sound quality issues to weakened doctor–patient rapport. She remarked that "the constellation was fine", but that "as a result of the bad sound, I had the tendency to get very close to the telephone, so I felt I was less with the doctor. I had to concentrate on the sound and then you lose a bit the rapport with the doctor." As a result of the sound quality, the patient found it tiring to listen to the interpreter. However, this did not affect the clarity of the information, according to the patient. What bothered the patient most in TI was getting distracted when the turns were too long. "When it's too long, I have the tendency not to focus on the doctor's answers anymore, you quickly think of other things, you are less 'in it.'" She added that "in between the talking, there is this empty space, like there is nobody, I don't know how to explain it, but afterwards you don't know who is going to talk". As for the interpreter, she mentioned that TI "has its limits", but emphasized that the interpreter's competence is of primary importance, saying "anyway, it's better to have a good interpreter over the phone than a bad one face-to-face".

VI-3

As far as their overall impressions were concerned, all participants were positive about VI. The interpreter mentioned that the "doctor and patient understood each other well" and were "on the same page". A negative aspect the interpreter mentioned had to do (once again) with a term she could not find, as a result of which she had to ask for clarification. Both the doctor and the patient praised the interpreter several times, for example, for being "very fast" and "professional". The patient added to her positive impression that, because the interpreter "translated" very quickly, there was a "real rapport with the doctor, because you don't have to think, has she understood me well? She does more than give the information, she also transfers exactly the emotions. In this way you can have more contact with the doctor." The communication was considered satisfactory by all participants, except for the moment of disconnection. The doctor mentioned this moment when she was asked about the possible negative aspects of the consultation, but also remarked that the issue was quickly solved. All participants considered the quality of care sufficient, as well as the seating arrangement (Figure 6) and technological conditions, apart from the moment the connection was lost.

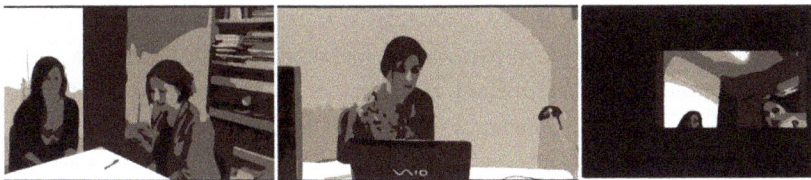

Figure 6. Seating arrangement in VI-3.

The doctor was enthusiastic about the seating arrangement in Series 3. According to her, the distance between her and the patient was very good this time (compared with Series 2, during which the participants were sitting too close to each other in the VI session, according to all participants). In this way, according to the doctor, she could have "a real conversation with the patient, also because the interpreter translated so quickly. In this way, I could keep contact very well with the patient." The patient found that she and the doctor were still seated rather close to each other, but that it was "okay". Surprisingly, the interpreter did not complain about the lack of visual access, even though she was only able to partly see the faces of the doctor and the patient, as the interpreter's screen recording shows.

Between VI and TI, all participants preferred VI. The interpreter commented: "I don't have experience with VI, except for the session today, but I have the impression it is comfortable. It is more pleasant to see your interlocutors. It is more personal." The doctor also mentioned the technological advantages, saying "between video and telephone [I prefer] video, mostly because the sound was better". She also had the impression that VI allowed for increased doctor–patient rapport in VI, compared to TI by saying "I have the impression that in VI, it is easier for the interpreter to get one's emotions across, apart from only by the intonation of your voice, as in TI. In VI, you can make a little bit more connection." Both the doctor and the patient made it very clear that their positive view of VI was very much related to the style and performance of the interpreter. "With this interpreter, VI is really an added value [compared with TI]", remarked the doctor. The patient confirmed this by saying that "with this interpreter, the video was as good as face-to-face. She translated so fast that it was as if I were alone with the doctor." The doctor also referred to the advantage of visual access by means of a webcam: "It is easy to see when somebody has finished [talking] and it makes it faster, you don't have to wait to make sure someone has finished, but you can see it." She also mentioned interactional issues: "Sometimes you start talking at the same time in TI. Here [in VI] that happens less and when it happens, it is less disruptive." However, it must be noted that, since there were only a few instances of overlapping speech in Series 3 in TI, the doctor may have been referring to her experiences with TI outside of the simulations.

7.2 Retrospective interviews

7.2.1 *Interpreter 1*

During the in-depth retrospective interview with Interpreter 1, the interpreter elaborated on the specific issues that had emerged in the first analysis and which were brought up by the researcher during the interview. However, as it turned out, many of the issues which were initially marked as salient appeared not to be extremely relevant to the research objectives. Moreover, the interpreter's remarks were sometimes contradictory and did not necessarily provide the information that the researcher was looking for. For example, when assessing her own performance, the interpreter was mainly preoccupied with assessing her ability to quickly find the right terms and seemed much less concerned with assessing her

Participant Perceptions 203

interactional skills, even after having been questioned about this explicitly. In addition, it was difficult to discern whether certain decisions were made consciously or not, since the interpreter did not really have a habit of reflecting on interpreting strategies in the same way interpreting studies scholars do. As a result, some of the requested clarifications did not generate satisfactory responses.

Given the above, despite the elaborate questioning, in the following synthesis of the interview, only comments which were relevant to the research aims are provided. The interview data are presented thematically, by means of four topics in total. The topics consist of the interpreter's negative remarks on VI (despite her general impression of satisfaction), the technical limitations of RI, the interpreter's notion of "increased neutrality" in RI and the interpreter's exclusion from the communication in VI.

Negative remarks versus satisfaction with VI

Despite her general impression of satisfaction with VI, in the post-simulation interviews, the interpreter's perception of this interpreting method was more negative in comparison to F2FI and TI. When we asked her to explain this, the interpreter told us that, contrary to what one would expect, to her, there are more similarities between TI and F2FI, than between VI and F2FI. According to the interpreter, the biggest problem with VI is the lack of full visual access. On her laptop screen, she only saw the primary participants' faces (or parts of these), instead of seeing the whole picture, including the environment. However, as she expressed it, "since VI imitates real life, interpreters must pretend to be in a F2FI situation" and, for example, "look up from time to time and pretend to make eye contact, even if this is not possible in VI". Otherwise, as stated by the interpreter, "there is no use of video". In TI, "this is less the case", since "people are more used to this way of communicating" and "act more naturally", the interpreter claimed. According to the interpreter, this makes VI more difficult than F2FI or TI.

Since the doctor and the patient had expressed contradicting comments in the post-simulation interviews concerning what was visible on their screens, the interpreter was asked what exactly she could see on her screen. According to her, only parts of the participant's faces were visible.

Unfortunately, since the screen recordings failed, the actual view could not be verified.

Technical limitations

When asked about the visibility of the primary participants in VI, the interpreter used the opportunity to complain about the technical limitations of TI as well. Contrary to the post-simulation interview, in the retrospective interview, the interpreter had many complaints about the technical aspects of the communication in TI. For example, she mentioned that using the speaker mode of the telephone made the communication less clear. In her day-to-day practice as an interpreter, she prefers that the primary speakers pass the receiver between them when it is their turn to speak, which makes it easier for her to "follow the person speaking". According to the interpreter, when the telephone is passed, the sound quality is better than in speaker mode.

"Increased neutrality"

In the post-simulation interview after VI, the interpreter had mentioned that the RI methods caused an "increased neutrality" in the relationship between the doctor and the patient, in the sense that "they were closer to one another without the physical presence of an interpreter". When she was asked to elaborate on this in the retrospective interview, the interpreter explained that "interpreters on a screen are like machines, they are there, but not really present". Generally speaking, according to the interpreter, the interpreter is "not really present" in RI, "only virtually". In her view, more distance can thus be created, as a result of which "neutrality is increased in remote interpreting". This was especially the case in VI, since in TI, according to the interpreter, "we are more likely to react naturally, as if we were just talking to another person, like in F2FI". Interestingly, this view is diametrically opposed to the patient's, who had complained in the post-simulation interview of the interpreter being "too obviously present" during VI-. It must be remarked that, even after the interpreter's explanations, her notion of "neutrality" remained rather vague.

Exclusion from the communication

In the analysis of miscommunication, some instances were observed in which the interpreter was excluded from the communication. This happened, for example, in VI, when the doctor and patient understood one another without the interpreter's intervention and the interpreter seemed to be behind (Excerpt 17). During the post-simulation interview after VI, the interpreter had mentioned feelings of detachment from the communication. She had also mentioned that, while practising VI, she had the feeling that she was "less involved in the communication" and that "VI seemed closer to conference interpreting than to community interpreting" by being "less social". Consequently, in the eyes of the interpreter, the communication was "less coherent" in VI than in the other interpreting methods. However, when asked whether she felt excluded from the communication when the patient and doctor had already understood each other before the interpreter had a chance to render the information, the interpreter answered no. According to her, it was "all for the better" if the doctor and patient had understood one another already before she had a chance to render the information, because "the whole idea of interpreting is that the patient and doctor understand each other".

7.2.2 Interpreter 2

The interview data are presented with a focus on three distinct topics: lack of note-taking, editorialization, and lack of terminology and language mixing.

Lack of note-taking

One of the important observations by the researcher in the exploratory analysis was that Interpreter 2 did not take any notes during any of the simulations, apart from the TI session, when she did take some notes sporadically. The explanation that the interpreter provided revealed much about her attitude towards interpreting, which may also explain other issues that were observed, such as omission. According to the interpreter, during the consultations, the turns were not extremely long and the content of the consultations was "not that complicated". Therefore, she did not feel it was necessary to take notes. She added that, in legal interpreting, for example, in a trial, interpreters are forced to be quite precise and must note down everything. By contrast, according to the interpreter, in medical interpreting, "you can ask the other participants in the consultation to repeat or clarify issues". In medical interpreting, as the interpreter explained, she feels "more free". The fact that the interpreter's renditions were in many cases less precise than the patient's and doctor's original utterances seems therefore to be supported by the interpreter's opinion that it not necessary to render all utterances when "their meanings can also be transferred with fewer words". This attitude towards interpreting led to a more summarizing interpreting style, which may also partly explain the large number of ME issues in Series 2, compared with Series 1 and 3. However, the interpreter did not seem to be aware of this, given her claim that "participants often have the habit of repeating themselves, saying the same thing in different words. [...] I get rid of some details then, but 90 or maybe 99 or even 100% of the message, I transfer."

Editorialization

As defined in Section 4.3.1, "editorialization" means that interpreters express their own opinion while rendering a participant's message, without the recipient of the message being aware of this (Flores et al., 2012). This happened three times in Series 2 (twice in the F2FI session and once in VI). In F2FI, the editorializations consisted of additions in the interpreter's renditions, specifying that a certain treatment was "very good" and "more practical". An example of this can be found in Excerpt 12, containing an addition by the interpreter to the doctor's message in VI. When the interpreter was asked to comment on these instances of editorialization, she answered that she was not aware of having added any information, but claimed to have just expressed the doctor's or patient's words in the way she had understood them: "When I added something, maybe I wanted to make something clear to the patient. Often you do not translate literally but almost explain the whole situation. I try to translate, but sometimes I just have to explain something, to make it clearer."

Lack of terminology and language mixing

In terms of the instances in which the interpreter was searching for terms, the interpreter mentioned that in F2FI, it was much easier to obtain help from the other participants than in the RI sessions. The interpreter explained: "In telephone interpreting, there is less interaction and you have to do more on your own." However, according to the interpreter, the help offered by the other participants sometimes also got "out of control". As an example of this, the interpreter recalled a moment when she could not think of a word and the doctor proposed a term in English. To the interpreter, this was the reason why she became confused and mixed up languages. When questioned about her relatively frequent language mixing, the interpreter explained that French was not her most active working language. In addition, she emphasized that her language mixing was a result of stress and "fatigue of the brain", which "occasionally happened" to her when she felt tense or tired, but never happens in her professional practice as an interpreter. According to the interpreter, the language mixing occurred as a result of stress caused by the experimental conditions.

7.2.3 Interpreter 3

The themes of this interview included perceived similarities between F2FI and VI, increased stress in TI, technical issues in TI and VI, and the interpreter's fast interpreting style. Since some of the themes touched on comparable phenomena, overlaps between the different topics could not be avoided.

Perceived similarities between F2FI and VI

During their individual interviews after the simulations, the patient and the doctor had stressed that the quality of VI was "nearly the same as

F2FI" because "the interpreting was so fast" and "the interpreter was excellent". When the interpreter was asked if she perceived any quality differences between F2FI and VI, she answered that according to her, there were hardly any. Looking back, she considered that her performance with VI was maybe the best one of the three interpreting methods. However, she also mentioned that this may have been related to the fact that it was the first simulation of the three and therefore she felt "very fresh and not yet tired". The interpreter spontaneously compared her performance in F2FI to the other two simulations. She stated having been "a bit nervous beforehand", but had the impression that "the first interpreting session went very well and that with the telephone interpreting, I had to write down a lot, because it is specific problems after all and no matters of everyday life at all". She added that in TI she was "more unhappy there, with the telephone in my hand and my pen as well, so there, I suffered a bit more, but for the rest I think it was okay, like the face-to-face session".

Increased stress in TI

Since the interpreter had mentioned increased stress in TI in the post-simulation interview and the video data showed her constantly manipulating her glasses during TI (something she did not do in the other sessions), she was asked to elaborate on this. The interpreter answered that she was not really aware of any increased stress: "I don't think so, or completely unconsciously, but I don't think so, yes my glasses, that happens when I can't read my own writing, but in face-to-face, I did not put on my glasses and I also wrote a lot […]. Maybe it was also linked to the subject, maybe it was the first subject, the one of the pelvic floor, maybe I was better prepared, or it was less difficult, or seemed more obvious to me … […]. It's not such an easy conversation, anyway, so you have to concentrate harder." She remarked again, like she did in the post-simulation interview following the TI session, that she had the impression that she always had to be quick, because of the lack of visual access. According to the interpreter, this may have triggered stress, without her being fully aware of it during the interpreting. "I just always had the impression that I had to make a quick note of something in order to be able to do it as quickly as possible." She added to this: "I'm not very good at notetaking and it's not very practical with the phone in my hand and I wasn't really stressed, but I did have the feeling that: it has to go faster here, I have to fill in the emptiness."

In her comments, the interpreter also indicated that with the speaker phone, interpreters have less time between turns (as compared with passing the telephone). "With the speaker mode [that was used], that [the empty spaces] is worse. If they pass each other the phone, then you have some time until the other one comes to the line, but here, with the speaker mode, you can really leave no blanks, no voids, you know?" The interpreter mentioned that she had always had the feeling that the other participants were waiting for her, "so it is important that I start interpreting at the right time" and that as a result of the lack of visual access, the other participants probably wondered what the interpreter was doing: "that, they don't like it, you know, they wonder what is going on with me". She pointed out that "in a face-to-face conversation, you can just take notes and then they will see this and understand, and then it's no problem", whereas, as she explained, "when you're on the phone, they think: okay, where is it?".

Technical issues in TI and VI

Contrary to the doctor and the patient, the interpreter was not bothered by the background noise during TI. However, when in the VI session, the connection was suddenly lost, she was very confused. The interpreter explained that she had no idea what to do in that moment. Initially, she thought it was part of the experiment, then she wondered if time was up already. "I didn't know very well what to do about it, if it was foreseen, if it was all over, should I go outside now? I stood up from my place for a while and I thought, hey, is it time already or something. I didn't realize it was a real technical defect."

Fast interpreting style

As mentioned in the analyses of the video data, Interpreter 3 had a very fast way of interpreting, which forced the participants to take relatively short turns. When asked if this was a deliberate strategy, the interpreter answered in the affirmative, although her answer was slightly contradictory. At first, she claimed to do this "perhaps, a little subconsciously". However, afterwards, she explained that she did this deliberately, "because the other one wants to know what something is about". She explained that she always starts interpreting when she has the impression that the turn is over, "when I think, okay, she has said what she has to say", and then renders the information to the patient as soon as possible. "Sometimes I do realize that something else is still coming up. Then I apologize and wait for the speaker to finish completely." However, as she explained, "I always try to pick it up as soon as she's spoken, immediately." The interpreter explained that her fast interpreting style is also a way of avoiding an overload of information in one turn: "Maybe that's a little for myself, to make it clear that it's been long enough." She also mentioned that she finds it better to chunk the information: "Personally, I also think it's better if short pieces are passed on, because the other person is just waiting all the time, if that person doesn't understand anything and doesn't know what it's all about, then the pieces shouldn't be too long." However, as she pointed out, chunking also helps the interpreter to process the information by adding: "Sometimes it's also just for my own comfort." Moreover, according to the interpreter, keeping the turns short is something she does automatically, even "a bit subconsciously". She explained this as: "I think I do this. I'm not going to interrupt the person, but if I have the impression, okay, he has spoken enough …." Although, according to the interpreter, an interpreter must be able to translate large pieces – which is also part of the training –, "if it takes too long, the interpreter should be saying 'hello, I'm here too!'"

CHAPTER 8

Conclusion and Discussion

This final chapter aims to wrap up and discuss the results from this research and answer the research questions, in light of findings in previous research on RI. It is structured as follows. First, the research objectives and questions are summarized (Section 8.1), followed by the main conclusions of the quantitative and qualitative analyses regarding miscommunication and interaction management (Sections 8.2 and 8.3). After that, the most important challenges of RI observed across the three interpreting methods and the three series are discussed (Section 8.4). This is followed by an outline of the implications of the research results for interpreting practice and training (Section 8.5), and of the limitations of this research (Section 8.6). To conclude, suggestions for future research on RI are provided (Section 8.7).

8.1 Summary research objectives and questions

The objective of this research was to investigate the quality of interpreter-mediated healthcare communication by comparing two remote interpreting (RI) methods – telephone interpreting (TI) and video interpreting (VI) – with face-to-face interpreting (F2FI). In healthcare settings, RI is increasingly being adopted as a means to improve access to healthcare and increase cost-efficiency. Medical studies involving experiments with interpreting over the telephone or by video link have reported predominantly positive results. However, these studies mostly reveal user satisfaction with the quality of care by using different interpreting methods rather than measure the potential impact of the different methods on the quality of interpreter-mediated healthcare communication. In interpreting studies too, most of the research on RI in medical contexts has focused on participants' perceptions. In other settings – such as conference interpreting, business interpreting and legal interpreting – , evidence-based research has demonstrated that the use of RI methods may influence interpreting performance. Nevertheless, to the best of my knowledge, no qualitative comparison of different interpreting methods together (F2FI, TI and VI) has been undertaken from the perspective of interpreting studies.

This research combined insights from several research perspectives (interpreting studies, medical studies and bilingual healthcare communication) to investigate the quality of interpreter-mediated healthcare communication. The investigation centred on the following five research questions:

1. Are there differences in quality in interpreter-mediated doctor–patient communication between the three interpreting methods under investigation (F2FI, TI, VI), as expressed by the number and nature of issues at the level of message equivalence and/or at the level of interaction?
2. Are there differences in interaction management in interpreter-mediated doctor–patient communication between the three interpreting methods F2FI, TI and VI, as expressed by the number and nature of repair and optimization strategies?
3. Is there a relationship between message equivalence issues and interactional issues?
4. Can possible differences in quality between the RI methods (TI, VI) and the F2FI method be attributed to environmental and/or technological factors?
5. Within the RI methods (TI, VI), are there benefits to the quality of the communication when using an audiovisual channel (VI) in comparison with an audio-only channel (TI)?

To answer these questions, a methodology consisting of a corpus of nine simulations of interpreter-mediated doctor–patient encounters was designed, involving three experienced interpreters, a professional gynaecologist and a simulated patient. All three interpreters performed their task in three different interpreting methods: (1) face-to-face interpreting (F2FI), (2) telephone interpreting (TI) and (3) video interpreting (VI). The collected data were transcribed, translated and annotated. Subsequently, a comparative qualitative analysis was conducted.

In this research, quality was defined as the achievement of effective communication in terms of reaching a mutual understanding between the patient and the healthcare provider (Meeuwesen et al., 2010). Since the effectiveness of interpreter-mediated communication was considered to depend on the interpersonal dynamics between the healthcare provider, the patient and the interpreter (Hsieh, 2017), the focus of the analysis was on the quality of the interaction between all three participants (doctor, patient, interpreter), taking into account the specific discourse environment of healthcare interpreting, as well as the multimodal character of communication.

The concept of quality was operationalized through the investigation of two closely related quality indicators in dialogue interpreting: miscommunication and interaction management. In order to formulate an answer to the research questions, a methodology was developed to assess interpreting quality – based on a combination of taxonomies used in previous empirical research in the fields of interpreting studies, discourse analysis and pragmatics (Table 7) – and discussed in detail in Section 4.3.

The collected data were analysed with a view to identifying possible differences in quality by studying miscommunication at the levels of message equivalence (ME) and interaction (IA), and the interaction management across the three interpreting methods and series, each involving a different interpreter (Interpreters 1, 2 and 3). The analyses also aimed to establish the impact of the remote conditions on the quality of interpreter-mediated communication by identifying potential relationships between ME and IA issues, as well as the influence of environmental and technological (ET) factors, as apparent from the investigation of concurring issues. In addition, between the two RI methods, the possible benefits of the audiovisual channel (VI) compared with the audio-only channel (TI) were examined.

In order to find out what caused miscommunication, how it occurred and how it was responded to interactionally by the participants, instances of miscommunication were analysed. These qualitative analyses focused on instances of concurrence that demonstrated most prominently the differences between the three interpreters and interpreting methods and were in line with Wadensjö's (1999) view that the outcome of the interpreting performance depends on the mutual relationships between the primary participants and between the primary participants and the interpreter, as well as on the participants' communicative styles.

The analyses of the video data was cross-referenced with two sets of participant interviews, one with each individual participant (doctor, patient and interpreter) immediately following the simulations, and one with each interpreter two weeks later, after a first analysis of the video data by the researcher.

8.2 Miscommunication

In all three series and interpreting methods, omission was the most frequent type of issue (Table 9). At the ME level (Table 8), differences in the number of issues across the three interpreting methods F2FI, TI and VI were found in two of the three series (Series 2 and 3), whereas in the other series (Series 1), the were hardly any differences in numbers across the three interpreting methods. This suggests that in Series 1, the was no direct influence of the remote conditions on quality at the level of message equivalence. This is in line with results reported by Wang and Fang (2019), which indicated that the interpreter participating in the simulations performed equally well in both F2FI and TI in terms of the accuracy of the interpretation. For VI, the results confirm findings from Balogh and Hertog (2012: 106) in the sense that, at the "product level" (which is similar to the message equivalence category in this research), "on the whole, the different forms of interpreting seemed to produce similar interpreting quality". However, the greater number of concurring issues in VI in Series 1, compared with F2FI and TI, do indicate that ME issues were more often linked to issues at the level of interaction (and technology and environment) in VI. Since most ME issues were omissions, this result

Conclusion and Discussion

corresponds with findings from previous research on VI, showing a correlation between omission and overlapping speech for this interpreting method (Braun & Taylor, 2012b).

The results from Series 2 show a higher number of ME issues in VI than in F2FI, which is in line with findings from Braun and Taylor (*ibid.*). However, between F2FI and TI, the differences in numbers were minimal in the same series, the percentage of ME issues that concurred with issues at the level of interaction and/or with technological and environmental issues was extremely low for all three interpreting methods, compared with Series 1 and 3, indicating few relationships between ME issues and issues at other levels. Yet, it must be noted here that the total number of ME issues in Series 2 was considerably higher in Series 2 than in Series 1 and 3. Despite the strict selection criteria determining the experience, training and professionalism of the interpreters, Interpreter 2 produced more than 1.5 times as many problematic ME issues as Interpreter 1, and even twice as many as Interpreter 3. Interpreter 2 also produced a higher number of false fluencies than Interpreter 1 and 3 and was also the only interpreter to express editorializations, that is, instances in which she expressed her own opinion on a source-text message, which happened twice throughout the three simulations she was involved in. Therefore, the increased occurrence of ME issues in Series 2 appeared to be linked more closely to interpreter's competence than to the interpreting method.

In Series 3, the remote conditions had no effect on the number of ME issues in VI, which was in fact significantly lower than in F2FI and TI. However, the number of ME issues was higher in TI than in the other two interpreting methods. At the same time, in Series 3, concurrence between issues at different levels was the lowest of all three interpreting methods in TI.

The great variation in the quantitative results at the ME level related to concurrence across the three interpreting methods in each series suggests that, overall, the remote conditions did not have a direct influence on the frequency of miscommunication and that reasons for the variation across the interpreters may rather be linked to their individual competence and interpreting style. These outcomes corroborate the results reported by Korak (2010) regarding the use of VI in healthcare settings, stating that the viability of VI depends greatly on the individual competence of the interpreters.

Interestingly, what all three series had in common was that the simulations with the highest average full-turn duration were also those in which the highest number of ME issues occurred. As previous research in interpreting studies has established, longer turns can cause memory overload, which can lead to a lower degree of accuracy (Balogh & Salaets, 2018). Of course, several factors determine turn duration. On the one hand, it can be the result of the interaction management by the interpreter, since they can influence the speed of the communication (Spinolo et al., 2018b: 17), as well as the duration of the turns, by deciding when to start the rendition. On the other hand, contextual factors also play a role in how interaction unfolds. For example, in the remote conditions, the interpreters had fewer opportunities to use backchannelling to indicate their intention of starting a rendition. Consequently, the interpreters may have been more or less forced to accept longer turns. Moreover, the extent to which interpreters actively intervene in the interaction management also depends on their personal views on appropriate professional interpreter behaviour, combined with experience, self-confidence and knowledge of the ways in which discourse processes unfold in specific settings. The effect of interpreters' and primary participants' interactional behaviour on communication will be further discussed as part of the qualitative analyses in Section 8.4.

As far as interactional issues are concerned, overlapping speech was clearly the dominant type of issue, the results from the quantitative analysis of the IA issues showing even fewer clear patterns than was the case for omission at the level of ME. In Series 1, the lowest number of IA issues was observed in F2FI and the highest in VI. This suggests that the remote conditions had an effect on the frequency of IA issues, particularly in VI. This effect also surfaced in the percentage of concurring issues, which was extremely high in VI compared with F2FI and TI in Series 1. The results for TI coincide with those from Wadensjö (1999) and Wang and Fang (2019), who reported increased numbers of IA issues in TI compared with F2FI. For VI, the findings are in line with Braun and Taylor (2012b), Balogh and Hertog (2012) and, for sign language interpreting (VRS), Warnicke and Plejert (2016).

Conclusion and Discussion

As was the case in Series 1, in Series 2, the percentage of concurring IA issues in VI was also extremely high compared with F2FI and TI, indicating a strong relationship between IA and ME issues and/or environment and technology (ET) issues. However, in Series 2, the remote conditions appeared to have no significant effect on the number of IA issues in VI. In fact, TI saw the highest number of issues of all three interpreting methods, indicating that the remote conditions made a slight impact, although the difference in numbers between TI and F2FI was extremely small.

No relationship between IA issues and issues at other levels was established in Series 3. In this series, the percentage of concurring IA issues was much lower than in Series 1 and Series 2 across all three interpreting methods. Moreover, as opposed to Series 1 and Series 2, the lowest percentage of concurring issues in Series 3 was observed in VI. It must be noted that, in Series 3, the total number of IA issues was twice as high as in Series 1 and 1.5 times higher than in Series 2. Moreover, there was quite a significant difference between the number of IA issues in F2FI and VI on the one hand, and in TI on the other. This appears to have been mainly the result of Interpreter 3's optimization of the communication in TI. As the qualitative analysis showed, Interpreter 3 deliberately slowed down the pace of the communication in TI by waiting longer to start her rendition after each turn, in order to prevent overlapping speech. This way of optimizing communication will be further explained in the discussion of the conclusions from the qualitative analyses in Section 8.4, which addresses the most important challenges of RI compared with F2FI.

8.3 Interaction management

To examine how participants dealt with communication breakdown, we examined the interaction management by looking into repair and optimization (RO) strategies. Across the different interpreting methods in each series, Series 1 and 3 showed comparable numbers as far as the number of repair and optimization strategies was concerned (Table 4). In both series, the lowest numbers of RO strategies were observed in F2FI and the highest numbers in VI. The results for TI confirm previous findings in TI research indicating a higher degree of meta communication (Oviatt & Cohen, 1992; Rosenberg, 2007; Wang, 2017), suggesting that interpreters were more active (or perceived themselves as more active) in the coordination of the interaction. For VI, an increase in "process overhead" (Olson et al., 1997: 170) was also established by (amongst others) Braun (2013, 2017), Braun and Taylor (2012b) and Warnicke and Plejert (2016).

On the contrary, Series 2 showed a very different pattern, with the highest number of RO strategies occurring in F2FI and the lowest in TI. Despite the lower numbers for the RI methods, the qualitative analyses showed that Interpreter 2 had more difficulties managing the interaction remotely, especially in VI. As was the case in all three series, additional IA issues often occurred during repair, which complicated the achievement of a mutual understanding. Moreover, whereas in F2FI the primary participants made efforts to collaborate in helping the interpreter find the right terminology, this was more difficult in TI and VI because of the limited possibilities of backchannelling between the primary participants and the interpreter. The primary participants also appeared less willing to support the interpreter in the RI conditions, whereas the interpreter mentioned in the interviews that she found it harder to initiate repair during RI.

In all three series, the technical conditions of RI complicated interaction management. In TI, the compromised sound quality of the speaker mode caused comprehension problems, which sometimes required repair. Moreover, environmental issues – such as noise from outside the room, from the street or from construction work in the building – complicated repair of miscommunication. Since the volume of the doctor's and the patient's voices was already reduced by the speaker mode, noise from outside forced the participants to fully concentrate on the speaker's voice, as a result of which they avoided gazing at each another and looked mostly at the telephone. They also positioned themselves closer to the phone and often frowned, indicating comprehension difficulties. Although this did not directly lead to miscommunication or repair most of the time, it did affect rapport-building between the participants, as they mentioned during the interviews and as became obvious from the analysis of the opening and closing sessions in the RI methods. The issue of rapport will be addressed more extensively in Section 8.4.3.

As far as the optimization of the communication is concerned, it was obvious that each of the three interpreters optimized the communication in ways that cannot be expressed by merely adding up numbers of optimization strategies. The ways in which the communication was optimized also related to interpreting style, competence and attitude, which in turn had an impact on the duration of the turns. For example, by giving the primary participants ample time to continue talking without interrupting them and therefore taking a rather passive stance, in TI, Interpreter 3 deliberately avoided overlapping speech. This more cautious way of communicating was also observed by Wadensjö (1999), who established longer turn transitions in TI compared with F2FI.

From the quantitative results related to miscommunication, concurrence, and repair and optimization strategies we can conclude that the influence of the remote conditions on each of these aspects of the communication was extremely varied across the series and interpreting methods. Although the data show that there were links between ME issues and IA issues, the extent of these relationships was quite different across the three interpreting methods and series. In fact, the impact of the remote conditions depended greatly on the ways in which the interaction was managed by all three participants in each individual series, as well as on the individual style and competence of the interpreters. Therefore, as we have seen, the impact of the remote conditions on the quality of the communication was quite different for each interpreter.

The analysis of overlapping speech in the corpus indicates that interaction management is more complex when RI methods are used, since these put constraints on the use of multimodal resources for backchannelling. Moreover, the technological and environmental conditions, such as the compromised volume of the speaker phone and the lack of visual access during TI, and the delay in sound and image, the reduced view and sound quality problems during VI had an effect on how overlapping speech unfolded and was managed. The qualitative analysis of the video data revealed that in the three series, certain phenomena occurring specifically in the remote conditions pointed to obvious differences in how miscommunication unfolded and how repair of miscommunication was carried out between the three different interpreting methods and the three interpreters. Surprisingly, as the results of the subjective data analysis showed, an increase in the number of IA issues and repair and optimization strategies (e.g. in Series 3) did not necessarily affect the participants' satisfaction with the quality of the interpreter-mediated communication or with the consultation in general.

A factor that appeared to play a decisive role in the positive assessment of the quality of interpreter-mediated communication seemed to be the smoothness of the communication, that is, the continuity of the communication flow. As long as there were not too many "hitches" inhibiting smooth interaction, whether these were the result of the participants' interactional behaviour, miscommunication, or the technological or other contextual conditions, the participants claimed that they were satisfied with the consultations. Even cases of communication breakdown (e.g. connectivity problems in VI) did not automatically affect the participants' satisfaction, provided that the breakdown was repaired quickly and efficiently.

8.4 Main communication challenges in RI

Below, the conclusions of the qualitative analyses of Series 1, 2 and 3 are summarized, comparing three features of the interaction that, in the data under investigation, posed the greatest challenges to successful communication when RI methods were used, as compared with the F2FI interpreting method. These include interactional behaviour (Section 8.4.1), smoothness of the communication (Section 8.4.2) and rapport (Section 8.4.3). Since these features are interrelated, there may be overlaps between the individual sections.

8.4.1 Interactional behaviour

As Pittarello (2012) argues, the ways in which participants organize interaction in terms of turn-taking and communication exchanges contributes to the success or failure of the interaction. For all three interpreting methods, the qualitative analyses of instances of concurrence and repair and optimization showed that the interactional behaviour of all three participants (doctor, patient and interpreter) was a crucial factor in determining the success of the interpreter-mediated communication. The analysis showed that the ways in which the interaction was managed when message equivalence issues or interactional issues occurred, played an important role in the achievement of a mutual understanding and the satisfaction of the participants with the consultation.

The most frequently observed and problematic issue resulting from interactional behaviour by all participants was overlapping speech. Overlapping speech by the interpreter mostly occurred a transition-relevance place (Jefferson et al., 1974) – that is, a possible end of a primary participant's turn – was in fact an intra-turn pause (Schegloff et al., 1977), when the interpreter mistook a pause for the end of a primary participant's turn. This resulted in a false start by the interpreter, causing overlapping speech. This type of issue did not cause communication breakdown in any of the F2FI consultations, although it did lead to omission and sometimes required repair. However, usually, repair was carried out efficiently in the F2FI sessions, heavily supported by backchannelling, especially gaze. Overlapping speech did not appear to be extremely problematic in TI either, given the participants' (especially the interpreters') more careful ways of communicating by leaving longer moments of silence in between the utterances and renditions. By contrast, in VI, overlapping speech frequently disrupted the communication flow due to the sound quality problems arising when two people spoke at the same time.

Overlapping speech by one of the primary participants during the interpreter's rendition also had a more disruptive effect on the communication in the remote conditions than in F2FI. This was clear from the interruptions in the form of reactive expressions of empathy (by the doctor) or emotion (by the patient). Examples of such reactive expressions are "yes, I can imagine" (uttered by the doctor) or "that is such a relief" (uttered by the patient). In all three interpreting methods, the interpreters omitted these reactive expressions most of the time in their renditions. This corroborates findings in research on F2FI medical interpreting by Anazawa et al. (2012), who report on the omission of minor words or brief phrases conveying empathic or validating signals between interlocutors, even by experienced interpreters. It also confirms findings from Krystallidou et al. (2018), who observed omission in the transfer of patients' emotional expressions and doctors' empathic responses in interpreters' renditions. According to Roy (2000), in face-to-face dialogue interpreting, the rendition of backchannelling responses is usually ignored by interpreters, since it is not possible for the interpreter to listen to two speakers and talk at the same time. Moreover, rendering this type of overlapping speech (i.e. a non-floor taking, reactive expression) could surprise the speaker and interrupt the speaker's train of thought (*ibid.*). Nevertheless, the analyses of the simulations demonstrated that omission of reactive expressions was partly compensated for by the backchannelling accompanying the reactive expressions (e.g. smiling, mutual gaze, intonation), providing the primary participants with information about intended meanings. However, only in F2FI did the interpreters have full access to backchannelling responses, which helped them to assess the relationship between the doctor and the patient and monitor comprehension and miscomprehension between the primary participants. By contrast, in TI, the interpreters obviously had no access to any of these visual cues and could only rely on auditive information, whereas in VI, visual access was limited because of a lack of full camera coverage of the primary participants. This made it more difficult for the interpreters to assess the degree of mutual understanding and construction of trust between the doctor and the patient. Between the two RI methods, especially in Series 1 and 2, the potential benefits of visual access in VI were for a large part outweighed by the disadvantages of VI, that is, sound quality problems due to overlapping speech and insufficient camera coverage.

The other most frequently observed cause for overlapping speech by the primary participants were interruptions due to requests for clarification. According to Wadensjö (1998), there are several strategies available for interpreters to manage this type of overlapping speech. Firstly, interpreters can interrupt the primary speaker and thus halt the primary speaker's turn, allowing the other speaker to continue (*ibid.*: 193). In the data under investigation, this situation never occurred, Secondly, interpreters can momentarily ignore a speaker's overlapping talk, keeping the utterance in

Conclusion and Discussion

memory, and continue rendering the turn they were interpreting at the moment they were interrupted. Subsequently, the "held" utterance can be rendered immediately following the end of the rendition. Thirdly, Wadensjö (*ibid.*) claims that interpreters can choose to ignore overlapping speech completely. Lastly, the interpreter can also momentarily ignore the overlapping talk and offer the primary speaker a turn upon finishing the rendition, or somehow indicate to the other speaker that a turn was attempted (*ibid.*: 194). Roy (2000) also claims that when overlaps occur, interpreters must react quickly and stop a speaker verbally or nonverbally, while considering factors such as message importance, participants' relationships, and relative status or authority. Like Wadensjö (1998), Roy (2000) also suggests that interpreters hold the utterance and recall it afterwards. This may be done when the interpreter deems the utterance not critical at the moment, or when the overlapping speech is short and easy to remember (*ibid.*: 89). However, as the scholar argues, sometimes interpreters no longer remember the utterance afterwards. The analysis of the simulations showed that finding the right moment to "catch up" with the interruption initiated by one of the speakers was indeed not an easy task for the interpreter. It frequently led to omission, even more so during the use of RI methods, which – as illustrated in a number of excerpts – severely restricted the use of subtle turn-taking hints by means of embodied communication such as eye gaze, body posture or gesture. These outcomes confirm the findings in VI by Braun (2004) indicating that interactional phenomena such as pauses, interruptions and backchannelling are often not perceived in the ways they were intended because of the timing difference caused by the delayed sound and image, however short this delay may be.

The findings for TI concerning interaction management are in line with those from Wadensjö (1999), who described problems with the synchronization of the interaction as a result of the different ways in which backchannelling functions in TI, compared with F2FI. In her opinion, even in face-to-face interpreting, the normal coordination of conversation between primary participants, supported by backchannelling, is partly lost because of the delay (in regular turn-taking) in between the primary participants' turns, since the interpreter's renditions are inserted in between. In TI, this feedback delay is even greater. As Wadensjö (1999: 305) argues, although experienced telephone interpreters can compensate for the reduced "communicative cues", the disadvantages for the interpreter increase when the sound quality is poor, or when participants speak in an inarticulate way, which was frequently the case in the simulations under investigation in this research study. This is consistent with the conclusions by Spinolo et al. (2018b), who claim that, in RI, the interpreter is the most disadvantaged party. However, the interview data of the current research also show that, in TI, the interpreters seemed to be much less bothered by the poor sound quality than the primary participants. In VI, then again, with the deterioration of the sound quality resulting from overlapping speech, the interpreters obviously were the most disadvantaged party.

8.4.2 Smoothness of the communication

The smoothness of the communication flow in terms of trouble-free turn-taking appeared to determine to a large extent the successfulness of the communication in terms of the participants' satisfaction with the interpreting methods. One of the aspects affecting smoothness was the pace of the communication. In all three series, the participants (especially the doctor and the patient) complained about the slowness of the communication in TI. Even though the average full-turn duration in TI was not in fact longer than in F2FI or VI in Series 1 and 2, the doctor and patient perceived the communication as slow. In Series 3, the perceived slowness was confirmed by the average full-turn duration, which was extremely long in TI compared with the F2FI and VI sessions. These findings are in line with Wadensjö's (1999), indicating that the deliberate avoidance of overlapping speech in TI made the communication less fluent.

Another interesting observation is that two of the three interpreters (Interpreters 2 and 3) took notes only during TI, whereas in F2FI and VI they hardly took any notes at all. According to González Rodríguez and Spinolo (2017: 245), taking notes during TI partially compensates for the "blindness" of the audio-only channel and helps interpreters to visualize the conversation. Interpreter 3 confirmed this during the in-depth interview that took place two weeks after the simulations. The note-taking in

TI, together with the extended time between the primary participants' turns and the interpreter's renditions, made the communication slower and the average turn duration longer than in F2FI and VI in Series 3. By not interrupting the speakers to ensure that they had finished speaking, Interpreter 3 successfully avoided overlapping speech. However, this success came at the expense of the participants' satisfaction. In Series 3, far fewer IA issues and repair strategies occurred in TI than in VI. However, the higher numbers of IA issues and repair strategies in VI did not affect the participants' satisfaction, which was just as high as in F2FI. The remark by one of the participants that "VI can be as good as F2FI, it all depends on the interpreter" is quite representative of the results in general. Interpreter 3 had a fast and efficient way of communicating. She often caused overlapping speech, but also monitored the communication extremely closely and stopped speaking immediately when she realized a primary participant had not finished her turn. In so doing, Interpreter 3 was able to maintain the communication flow, despite the occurrence of interactional issues. This monitoring of the interaction is critical for successful communication. As previous research has shown, interpreter self-regulation – which can relate to affect, behaviour, cognition and context – is essential to maintain or increase alignment with the interaction and the goal of the interpreting performance (Herring, 2019).

Interpreter 3's extremely fluent way of interpreting contrasted quite radically with the style of Interpreter 2, who often seemed insecure, as expressed by her numerous hesitations during her renditions, when she was looking for the appropriate terms or the appropriate way of formulating messages. This made the communication management rather inefficient and affected the primary participants' interactional behaviour. The doctor in particular seemed annoyed with the hesitations and slow communication rhythm at times, mainly when the RI methods were being used, delaying the pace of the communication even more. For example, in TI, which the participants already perceived as slow, the doctor seemed extremely anxious to finish the consultation and showed her exasperation by hanging up the receiver and not letting the interpreter finish saying goodbye. Moreover, in both TI and VI (compared with F2FI), the doctor and the patient seemed less inclined to help the interpreter to find the appropriate terms (see Excerpt 23 for an example). In Series 2, it seemed that when the communication flow was less smooth, the participants seemed less willing to help the interpreter find the right terms, even at the expense of their own mutual understanding. This may be related to the fact that in the RI methods, the less direct way of communicating and limited access to backchannelling make collaboration between participants more complicated. Collaborative efforts to achieve a mutual understanding even had an opposite effect in RI, when the regular turn-taking system – in which the interpreter has every turn after the primary speaker – was disturbed and overlapping speech caused sound quality problems. For example, in Series 1 (Excerpt 19), the doctor wanted to help the patient find the name of the medication that she was using, but the doctor was in fact taking the turn of the interpreter, causing overlapping speech and a disruption of the communication. While the doctor and patient quickly arrived at a mutual understanding, the interpreter was excluded from the communication and expressed nonverbal signs indicating uncertainty and stress.

Another factor affecting the smoothness of the communication in RI was the limited possibilities for backchannelling. As Spinolo et al. (2018b: 20) state,

> a simultaneous access to multiple sensory inputs (visual, vocal, or even tactile and olfactory) provides the interpreter (and primary participants as well) with a very wide range of expressive resources that can positively contribute to a better understanding of the interlocutor's role in the conversation and the relationship among them, as well as offer an insight into the setting, context, symmetries/asymmetries of power, or any other nonverbal clue that might be missing or only partially available in remote interpreting.

As observed for the RI methods, it was nearly impossible for the interpreters to monitor mutual understanding between the primary participants by assessing subtle backchannelling exchanges between them. Moreover, the use of backchannelling between the interpreter and the primary participants was equally difficult, which rendered the synchronization of the interaction more challenging, especially when repair was needed. According to Gumperz (2005), successful interaction depends on correctly inferring the speaker's intention and continuously verifying if one's message is received as intended. Obviously, in RI, the reduced options for backchannelling complicated making this inference. Consequently, the communication flow in the RI sessions was often less smooth, especially in VI, since the technical conditions did not allow for simultaneous speech and overlapping speech frequently caused sound distortion. Moreover, when repair of miscommunication was needed, this often invoked further IA issues and/or omission of content, which in turn required repair. These chains of repair were only observed in VI.

The smoothness of the communication was furthermore affected by the professional custom of "translating everything" (as prescribed by a large number of professional interpreters' codes). In F2FI, this is already a challenging task, since it delays the communication. However, in RI, where the delay in communication is greater, applying this professional norm can seriously disrupt the communication flow. As we have seen (e.g. Excerpt 19), when the interpreter insisted on "translating everything" in VI, including meta communication (e.g. informing one primary participant that the other participant had asked a question), this made the communication less efficient. When the patient was trying to remember the name of a certain medication and the doctor helped her by suggesting the name, they quickly arrived at a mutual understanding. However, since the interpreter did not have full access to the participants'' multimodal behaviour, she could not really follow the communication between them. As a result of the interpreter's decision to translate each turn, she actually fell behind. Moreover, since the exchanges were accompanied by overlapping speech (causing sound quality problems in VI), smooth communication was undermined even further (e.g. Excerpt 22).

In other words, in some cases, "translating everything" made the communication inefficient, especially when the primary participants started to "help" each other or the interpreter. In this type of situation, interpreters must be aware of the constructive character of medical consultations, which implies that the primary participants show collaborative behaviour to arrive at a mutual understanding. Therefore, as became apparent from the detailed analyses, especially in VI, the interpreter may manage the interaction more efficiently by adopting a more flexible approach. Depending on the situation, the interpreter must make a judgement about how important it is at that moment to apply the professional code strictly, or determine whether it may wiser to temporarily deviate from the principle of translating everything in order to maintain a smooth communication flow.

Of course, making such a decision is also influenced by the interpreter's professional self-concept. The notion of professional self-concept, referring to professional interpreters' understanding of their own abilities and their responsibilities towards the stakeholders involved in the interpreting process, was originally conceived for conference interpreters by Andres (2011, in Englund Dimitrova & Tiselius, 2016). Englund Dimitrova and Tiselius (2016) complemented this definition with the notions of self-concept as defined for translators by Muñoz-Martín (2014: 28), who described self-concept as "awareness of the situation, of oneself and of self-efficacy, which all shape motivated decision-making". It is evident that interpreters with a well-developed self-concept are aware of the impact of their behaviour as interpreters and as participants in the communication. These interpreters are also more likely to be successful in performing their tasks while using RI methods than interpreters with a less developed professional self-concept.

At the same time, the interactional behaviour by the primary participants indicated little awareness of the fact that the interpreter could not always follow the communication between them. This confirms the results by Hansen (2020) and Hansen and Svennevig (2021) for VRI in healthcare settings, who demonstrate that the primary participants (together in one location) often do not realize that the interpreter (connected remotely) does not share the same visual ecology and, as such, misses out on important multimodal cues for interaction management. These results shows how important it is for all participants to be aware of the limitations of the communication media used, especially with regard to multimodal cues, and the effects of their interactional behaviour.

8.4.3 Rapport

As discussed earlier in this work, doctor–patient rapport is an important part of medical encounters that promotes a mutual understanding between participants in therapeutic encounters. In interpreting studies as well as in medical studies, the development of doctor–patient rapport is considered one of the prerequisites for effective communication. Studies in bilingual healthcare (Hsieh & Hong, 2010) and in interpreting studies (Krystallidou et al., 2018) have shown that the interpreter's performance can have significant implications for the clinical, emotional and empathic aspects of care. By omitting elements from the source text related to empathy or emotions, interpreters can harm interpersonal relationships between primary participants. As Iglesias-Fernández (2010) argues, a large part of the achievement of a mutual understanding and rapport-building is carried out by means of nonverbal communication. This implies that, in RI conditions, which lack or reduce access to visual cues, rapport-building may be at risk. Since the doctor and the patient were in the same location in the simulations under investigation in this research, the nonverbal exchanges between them were accessible to both of them. However, as discussed in the previous section, the interpreters could not receive such cues with the source text utterances, since they had no full access to the backchannelling between the primary participants, which weakened their understanding of the messages. Furthermore, this jeopardized the rapport between interpreters and the primary participants, since it partly excluded the interpreters from the communication when the RI methods were used, as demonstrated by the qualitative analyses of the simulations.

Another aspect related to rapport is interaction management. The detailed analyses of interaction management in Chapter 6 showed that, especially in Series 1 and 2, repair was carried out less smoothly in RI, making the interpreter more visible as a participant. Previous research on dialogue interpreting has reported that, when the interpreter is too present in the foreground, this may harm the rapport between the doctor and the patient (Mason, 2009). The impression that the interpreter was more present in RI than in F2FI, because of the more frequent communication breakdowns, was also voiced in the participant interviews, most explicitly by the patient, especially in VI. By contrast, in one of the series (Series 3), no such complaints were made by the primary participants after the VI session. Instead, both the doctor and the patient praised the interpreter's competence and emphasized that "with a good interpreter", there were very few differences between VI and F2FI, even if they preferred F2FI. The preference for F2FI confirms findings from medical studies summarized by Azarmina and Wallace (2005), Corey et al. (2017) and Masland et al. (2010), who also reported on a general preference for F2FI.

Of course, studying the participants' perceptions was the most direct way of knowing whether rapport-building was different in the three interpreting methods under investigation. Although the participants were not directly questioned about rapport, their remarks on the quality of healthcare, communication, seating arrangement and technology revealed that, in their experience, rapport-building between the doctor and the patient was affected in both TI and VI. This is in line with the findings from some of the medical studies, for example, Price Leemann et al. (2012). In the VI sessions, the seating arrangement for the doctor and the patient also influenced the participants' perceptions and prompted them to express negative comments related to rapport. Whereas in Series 1, the interpreter saw only part of the doctor's and the patient's bodies, in Series 2, the primary participants were seated so closely together that the interpreter had the impression that they were friends. According to Interpreter 2, this made it difficult for her to adopt a professional approach. The doctor and the patient also claimed not to be satisfied with this arrangement. According to the doctor, it undermined her authority as a doctor. By contrast, in Series 3, in which all participants claimed to be as satisfied with F2FI and VI, the recordings of the interpreter's screen show that, in fact, the interpreter and the primary participants had a very limited view of each other. Yet, none of the participants expressed any negative remarks on this, which may indicate that users focus more on the disadvantages of technological issues when they are less satisfied with the communication in general.

Apart from the seating arrangement, the participants also uttered complaints about environmental issues in RI, such as external noise, which compromised sound quality, especially in TI. However, the biggest threat to rapport-building were the technological conditions of the RI methods, about which the primary participants in particular voiced the most negative remarks. Whereas as all participants complained about the sound quality in TI, the patient and the doctor also mentioned detachment from the conversation, mostly as a result of the slowness of TI. This detachment, especially in TI, was also obvious from the direction of the participants' gaze. Both the doctor and the patient commented that they felt they had to concentrate on the sound so much that they mostly looked at the telephone instead of at each other. This was slightly better in VI, where despite frequently gazing at the screen, the participants gazed more often at each other than they had in TI. However, in VI, feelings of detachment from the communication were reported by the patient, most prominently in Series 1, where communication breakdown was highest in VI compared with F2FI and TI.

In the discussion of participants' perceptions, attention should also be paid to the difference in perspectives of the individual participants. As reported in previous research on remote conference interpreting, there are often differences between interpreters' and clients' perceptions of performance quality (Andres & Falk, 2009). As Mouzourakis (1996) argues, interpreters and non-interpreters have different views on quality. Other research into subjective assessments of interpreting quality in interpreting studies also claimed that clients of interpreting performances are not necessarily in a position to assess an interpreter's performance (Shlesinger, 2007). Moreover, clients tend to be less rigorous about quality than interpreters (Braun, 2013). Based on the data analysis from the present research, these findings can be complemented by the observation that expectations also differed between the clients themselves, in this case the doctor and the patient. The patient was rather critical in her opinion of the RI methods, especially with regard to rapport. For her part, the doctor took into account the financial and logistical advantages of the RI methods (especially VI) and was, therefore, more inclined to accept potential shortcomings.

Among the more general trends observed in all nine simulations was gaze direction in TI. Whereas in F2FI and VI, the primary participants often engaged in mutual gaze (although considerably less in VI than in F2FI), in TI, they mostly stared at the telephone or away from each other. In so doing, they undermined rapport-building, which may have contributed to the reduced satisfaction of the primary participants with this interpreting method. Moreover, in VI, none of the three interpreters ensured that the videoconferencing set-up was suitable by ensuring that all participants, including the interpreter herself, were visible on the screen before starting the actual consultation, during the so-called "pre-opening" (Amato, 2018: 79). Interpreter 1 adjusted her screen only at the request of the doctor but did not ask the doctor to do the same, then complained afterwards that her view of the primary participants was extremely limited. When asked for an explanation, Interpreter 1 responded that she felt that there was no time for this and that she had to start interpreting immediately. As a result of this lack of initiative from the interpreters to establish viable working conditions for VI with the primary participants, the interpreters had an extremely limited or even distorted view of the doctor and patient, although not all the interpreters seemed to be bothered by this to the same extent. The interpreters' failure to create appropriate conditions probably results from their lack of experience with VI and is, therefore, also linked to the interpreter's professional self-concept. Since the lack of visual cues in turn hampered rapport-building between the interpreter and the primary participants, the remote conditions indirectly affected rapport in VI during the opening management. Therefore, in RI, especially in the opening phase of VI, a more proactive approach by the interpreter is needed.

The effect of the remote conditions on rapport-building was also visible in the opening and closing management of the consultations. As we have seen, these phases are crucial for the participants to establish and confirm rapport-building (Braun & Davitti, 2018; Heath, 2004/1986). Another matter that must be kept in mind in the management of the opening phase are the differences in RI and F2FI related to nonverbal input. Whereas in F2FI, time is needed for the participants to enter the room, sit down, etc., in RI, for the interpreter, the interaction starts immediately. As a result, mutual identification cannot be negotiated in the same way as in F2FI (Spinolo et al., 2018b: 19). Therefore, especially in RI, it is important for interpreters to take the necessary time to introduce themselves and negotiate the basic rules for the communication with the primary participants. This is also recommended in, for example, the *Handbook of Remote Interpreting* (González Rodríguez, 2018).

As far as the closing phase is concerned, differences were observed in two of the three series between the two RI methods and F2FI. In both TI and VI, the consultations were closed much more hastily and abruptly than in F2FI. Moreover, the participants all looked eager to end the RI sessions, as expressed by their quick goodbyes, causing non-problematic overlapping speech. During the closing of the TI session in Series 2, the doctor even hung up the phone while the interpreter was still speaking, showing that she was anxious to finish the consultation (Section 6.2.2). As Braun and Davitti (2018: 133) argue, a smooth and effective closing ensures that the rapport that was built during the interaction is not jeopardized. The rushed closings observed during the RI methods, notably in Series 1 and 2, can therefore be considered a negative effect on the establishment of rapport, especially because specialized consultations, such as the simulation under investigation, are likely to be extended over various encounters between the patient and the doctor. Yet, a short closing did not necessarily mean that rapport-building was at risk. In Series 3, the closings were fast without being hasty, which was very much the result of the style of Interpreter 3, who focused on keeping the communication flow constant. Despite the interpreter's slower pace of turn-taking in TI, no nonverbal or verbal behaviour by the primary participants indicating irritation or tiredness was observed in any of the closings in Series 3. Another factor that played a role in these more constructive closings of the RI sessions in Series 3 was time. When the duration of the simulations in Series 1 turned out to be quite long and exhausting for the participants, decisions were made to reduce the approximate consultation time from 20 to 15 minutes. In Series 2, the closing was still rushed. However, in Series 3, the fast interpreting style reduced the duration of the consultation altogether, as a result of which the participants seemed less tired. These observations imply that the quality of remote interpreter-mediated healthcare communication would benefit from being limited in duration.

8.5 Implications for interpreter practice and training

Despite the mixed results of the quantitative analyses of miscommunication, concurrence, and repair and optimization, the thematic summary of the qualitative analysis indicates that, across the three series, some more general tendencies related to the specific characteristics of the RI methods could be observed. However, since the frequency of miscommunication seemed to be more closely linked to average full-turn duration instead of being a direct result of the remote conditions, the impact of the remote conditions on the quality of interpreter-mediated communication can be considered primarily indirect. Nevertheless, a direct influence of technological factors was observed, for example, in the form of sound quality issues or loss of internet connection, although the impact of technological and environmental factors was also in large part determined by the way the interaction was managed by all three participants, particularly the interpreter. Besides appropriate technological and environmental conditions, the successfulness of the interpreter-mediated communication depended greatly on the individual interpreters' competence, style and self-concept, as well as on the interactional behaviour displayed by all participants, which influenced the smoothness of the communication and rapport-building.

These results are extremely useful to all users of RI services, first and foremost to interpreters. When the interpreters who participated in the simulations were asked if they were satisfied with their performance in the post-simulation interviews, they focused mostly on the linguistic issues that they experienced as problematic. However, they hardly seemed to reflect on their achievements at the level of interaction management. Especially when RI methods are used, interpreters should be taught about potential interactional communication issues and useful coping strategies.

Developing interpreters' professional self-concept and self-monitoring would also help interpreters to establish basic rules of communication and appropriate RI working conditions with the participants before each RI assignment. Moreover, a more developed self-concept, based on strategic decision-making, would support interpreters in intervening more actively and more consciously in the management of the interaction. In so doing, they could contribute to minimizing the risks of reduced communication quality.

The insights into RI generated in this work are also useful for interpreter training. In training, more attention should be paid to the different interpreting methods that future interpreters will work with as soon as they enter the labour market, where the use of RI is much more established than it is in interpreting training. This preparation can consist of identifying the specific characteristics and possible pitfalls of RI methods and integrating

Conclusion and Discussion

these methods into interpreter training. For example, future interpreters can prepare for real-life interpreting practice by means of RI simulations, which can help them to develop a proactive attitude to minimizing negative side effects of RI.

The same goes for dialogue interpreters who are not familiar with the different RI methods. Research-based training initiatives are increasingly being developed, for example, the training project "Shift in Orality", which demonstrates the increasing importance of RI training in community settings. RI training for interpreters and users of interpreting services at regional levels – such as the training offered by the public service interpreting and translation service Atlas, in Antwerp, Belgium, which integrates research-based input in their training ("Working with a video interpreter"[1]), – are to be welcomed if we want to continue to improve the quality of communication with RI methods.

As the present research has amply demonstrated, awareness of the effects of one's interactional behaviour is also extremely important for patients and healthcare providers. Since all participants contribute to arriving at a mutual understanding and smooth, cooperative interaction, the participants' awareness of the effects of their interactional behaviour is crucial for the successfulness of the communication.

Insight into the challenges that RI methods pose for the quality of communication are also useful to other stakeholders involved, for example, digital platforms providing RI services. These services can take knowledge about the challenges of RI into account in the development of appropriate communication channels that support high-quality RI. In addition, healthcare policy makers can benefit from insights into the pros and cons of RI methods when deciding on their institutions' communication policy concerning language-mediation for foreign-speaking patients, which at the same time contributes to the development of truly inclusive and accessible public services for all citizens.

Lastly, the results also show that, especially in community settings, more investments should be made in high-standard hardware and software for TI and VI, in order to better control the technical quality of RI

---

1 <https://www.atlas-antwerpen.be/nl/agenda/werken-met-een-videotolk-2>.

communication. Despite the rapid improvement of the quality of videoconference technology and equipment in the last few years, the occurrence of technical issues such as connectivity problems is inevitable and must be taken into account. Therefore, when RI is used on a larger scale, continuous technical support service should be available. Moreover, stakeholders should strive for minimum standards for the use of RI in community settings and follow the example of the professional organization of conference interpreters AIIC, which implemented ISO standards for remote conference interpreting as early as 1998 (Section 2.1). The establishment of minimum technical requirements would also help to move interpreters away from their position as the most disadvantaged party in RI.

8.6 Limitations of this study

The findings of this study have to be considered in light of some of its limitations. In this final section, I discuss three methodological and four more general limitations.

As far as methodology is concerned, a first limitation relates to research design. Obviously, as stressed in Chapter 4, the sample was obviously too small to draw any significant quantitative conclusions through generalizations. The quantitative analysis primarily served as a way of counting the instances of miscommunication and repair and optimization, and identifying concurrence. However, a balance had to be found between presenting the overall picture of the results and the individual analyses, which needed to be sufficiently detailed. This turned out to be quite challenging, especially given the richness of the data from the three cameras, to which screen captures were added for Series 2 and 3. Because of the comparative research design, multimodal aspects could be taken into account only to a certain degree, leaving little space for more granular multimodal analyses. Nevertheless, following Mason (2000: 229–230), the research design was appropriate for "showing regularities of behaviours and co-occurrence of various features". Moreover, the collected data can still be used for more detailed, multimodal analyses, as will be discussed in the suggestions for future research in Section 8.7.

A second limitation is the use of simulations. I chose to work with simulations to increase the comparability of the three interpreting methods under investigation. However, the artificial nature of the simulations, combined with the obtrusiveness of the three cameras used to record them and the presence of the researcher as an observer, may have influenced the interaction. Therefore, the results of the analyses of the simulations may not apply to authentic data in the same ways. Nevertheless, it would be highly interesting to verify the findings of this research by analysing similar authentic data to investigate correspondence between simulated and authentic data, as proposed in the suggestions for further research in Section 8.7.

A third limitation is related to the practical implementation of the simulations, in particular the seating arrangement and the technological conditions. As far as the seating arrangement is concerned, I experimented with different constellations in VI, finding none fully satisfactory because the participants were either partly out of camera view or seated too close to each other. Moreover, despite the moveable display of the tablet in VI, the participants never moved this device. Similar problems have been reported in previous research, for example, in Braun and Taylor (2012b), Braun (2017) and Licoppe and Veyrier (2017). So far, no VI research has generated convincing results on the ideal constellation of the primary participants in VI. In addition, at the time of the simulations in 2016, wide-angle webcams were not as readily available on the market as today. With regard to the technological conditions, leaving the choice of wearing a headset in VI to the interpreters did not turn out to be the best possible solution. None of the interpreters chose to wear a headset, and the sound in VI turned out to be compromised. Therefore, it would have been better to make the use of a headset mandatory.

In TI, in line with previous research by Ko (2006), a speakerphone was used – as opposed to passing the telephone between the primary participants. However, this compromised sound quality, which turned out to be quite an obstacle to comprehension between the participants. Since the primary participants had to concentrate on listening carefully, they gazed at the telephone instead of making eye contact with each other, thus affecting rapport-building.

Some more general limitations to be acknowledged were more or less beyond my control. Firstly, the dedicated videoconferencing platform that I had planned to use (and tested beforehand) failed during the implementation of Series 1, so I had to resort to Skype video calling. Secondly, due to failure of the capture option of the interpreter's screen in Series 1, the interpreter's view of the primary participants could not be verified. Thirdly, the relocation before Series 2 and 3 of the university campus in which the Series 1 simulations had taken place was unfortunate. Although (in theory) the Wi-Fi conditions were comparable in the two buildings, since they were both served by the same university network, the local conditions (differences in the two buildings' construction, noise, etc.) caused slight variations in the technological conditions between Series 1 and Series 2 and 3. A fourth factor that was beyond our control was related to the availability of the simulated patient. The simulated patient participating in Series 1 informed me the day before the implementation of Series 2 and 3 that she was not able to join the simulations and instead suggested that we work with a colleague who would replace her. To mitigate the effect on the comparability of the simulations, the substitute simulated patient received a thorough briefing by the first one and watched the videos of Series 1 to familiarize herself with the simulations. In so doing, the effects of the replacement on the comparability of the data were minimized.

8.7 Suggestions for future research

This research has contributed to the increasingly growing body of knowledge on RI in specific settings, namely the context of healthcare communication. As the body of research on RI continues to expand, it will be interesting to use the results and methodology of this research as a basis for further investigations into the topic. In this section, we list three main suggestions for future research.

Conclusion and Discussion 239

Firstly, one of most important results, that is, the finding that the smoothness of the communication is an important factor in the successfulness of interpreter-mediated communication, can be explored in greater detail. Such an investigation could explore the specific aspects that determine the smoothness of the communication, for example, average turn duration, the duration of turn transitions and the ways in which these are achieved. Since the results of this research suggest a relationship between longer average turn duration and increased miscommunication, it would be highly interesting to further explore the effects of increased turn duration on cognitive load in F2FI and RI methods, for example, by means of experimental (comparative) research.

Secondly, it would be interesting to compare the results of this research with findings from similar research in different settings, using different language combinations, to establish similarities and differences in the effect of the use of RI and investigate to what extent the observed phenomena were related to specific contextual characteristics. In addition, the methodology of this study assessing interpreter-mediated communication in healthcare settings could be applied to investigate authentic data, in order to establish the extent to which the analyses of simulated data correspond to the analyses of authentic data. Moreover, this work has suggested that the behaviour of the users of RI is one of the factors that can be adapted. Therefore, longitudinal research in the field of remote healthcare interpreting is needed to study the effects of the use of RI and RI training over extended periods of time. Such long-term studies could address – besides the quality of the communication – manifold factors related to RI, such as interpreters' working conditions and remuneration, and interpreters' ethics. Apart from longitudinal studies, research collecting larger amounts of data could generate more representative results to establish the effect of the remote conditions on the quality of interpreter-mediated communication.

Thirdly, continuing the investigation of human factors interacting with technology could play an important role in managing the technological turn in interpreting and ensuring the responsible use of interpreter-mediated remote communication. Today, the use of RI methods is part of the daily reality for most professional interpreters. However, the appropriate implementation of RI is still much discussed in interpreter practice and research (Licoppe & Veyrier, 2017). It is evident that, as far as RI in DI settings is concerned, specifically in healthcare contexts, more research on the interaction between humans and technology is needed. Therefore, Moser-Mercer's (2005b: 75) call for a focus on human factors in RI research is still highly relevant today:

> While cost and effort necessary to ensure high-quality remote interpreting set-ups are certainly still not negligible, they are likely to decrease as equipment becomes less expensive and technical support staff become more experienced. Human factors then emerge as one of the most important issues to be explored in remote interpreting.

As a final remark, it must be stressed that, despite the shortcomings of RI that emerged in the data analyses, the results of this research are rather positive. As we have seen, the challenges that RI poses for the quality of interpreter-mediated communication depend mostly on factors that can be manipulated to some extent, such as providing viable technological and environmental conditions. As this study has shown, the degree to which these challenges pose a risk to quality is in large part determined by the competency and self-efficacy of the interpreter and the behaviour of the participants, who can all be guided and trained in anticipating and overcoming potential communication problems associated with RI methods.

Based on the results of the current study, I can agree with claims made in previous research (Andres & Falk, 2009; Braun, 2012) that with high-quality equipment and experienced and trained interpreters, many of the disadvantages of RI can be overcome. Given the willingness of participants to collaborate to arrive at a mutual understanding, as well as the progress of technology, RI can be considered a viable interpreting method – alongside F2FI –, provided that its specific characteristics are acknowledged and taken into account.

Bibliography

AIIC. (2000). Guidelines for the use of new technologies in conference interpreting. *Communicate!* March–April 2000. <http://www.aiic.net/ViewPage.cfm?page_id=120>.

Albl-Mikasa, M., & Tiselius, E. (Eds). (2022). *The Routledge Handbook of Conference Interpreting*. London: Routledge. doi: 10.4324/9780429297878

Alley, E. (2012). Exploring remote interpreting. *International Journal of Interpreter Education*, 4(1), 111–119.

Altman, J. (1994). Error analysis in the teaching of simultaneous interpreting: A pilot study. In S. Lambert & B. Moser-Mercer (Eds), *Bridging the Gap: Empirical Research in Simultaneous Interpretation* (pp. 25–38). Amsterdam: John Benjamins. doi: 10.1075/btl.3.05alt

Amato, A. (2018). Challenges and solutions: Some paradigmatic examples. In A. Amato, N. Spinolo, & M. J. González Rodríguez (Eds), *Handbook of Remote Interpreting: Research Report Shift in Orality Erasmus + Project: Shaping the Interpreters of the Future and of Today* (pp. 79–98). <https://www.shiftinorality.eu/es/resources/2018/05/11/shift-handbook-remote-interpreting>.

Amato, A., & Spinolo, N. (2018). Introduction. In A. Amato, N. Spinolo, & M. J. González Rodríguez (Eds), *Handbook of Remote Interpreting: Research Report Shift in Orality Erasmus + Project: Shaping the Interpreters of the Future and of Today* (pp. 79–98). <https://www.shiftinorality.eu/es/resources/2018/05/11/shift-handbook-remote-interpreting>.

Anazawa, R., Ishikawa, H., & Kiuchi, T. (2012). The accuracy of medical interpretations: A pilot study of errors in Japanese-English interpreters during a simulated medical scenario. *Translation & Interpreting*, 4(1), 1–20.

Anderson, A., O'Malley, C., Doherty-Sneddon, C., Langton, S., Newlands, A., Mullin, J., Fleming, A. M., & Van der Velden, J. (1997). The impact of VMC on collaborative problem solving: An analysis of task performance, communicative process, and user satisfaction. In K. Finn, A. Sellen, & S. Wilbur (Eds), *Video-mediated Communication* (pp. 133–155). Mahwah, NJ: Lawrence Erlbaum.

Anderson, L. (1994). Simultaneous interpretation: Contextual and translation aspects. In S. Lambert & B. Moser-Mercer (Eds), *Bridging the Gap: Empirical Research in Simultaneous Interpretation* (pp. 101–120). Amsterdam: John Benjamins. doi: 10.1075/btl.3.11

Anderson, R. B. W. (1976/2002). Perspectives on the role of interpreter. In R. W. Brislin (Ed.), *Translation: Applications and Research* (pp. 208–228). New York: Gardner Press.

Andres, D., & Falk, S. (2009). Remote and telephone interpreting. In D. Andres, & S. Pöllabauer (Eds), *Spürst Du wie der Bauch rauf runter?: Is everything all topsy turvy in your tummy? Fachdolmetschen im Gesundheitsbereich/Health Care Interpreting* (pp. 9–27). Munich: Martin Meidenbauer.

Andres, D. (2011). Ein integrativ konzipiertes Dolmetschprozessmodell. *Studia Universitatis Babes-Bolyai: Philologia, 1*, 81–103.

Andres, D., & Falk, S. (2009). Remote and telephone interpreting. In D. Andres & S. Pöllabauer (Eds), *Spürst Du wie der Bauch rauf runter?: Is everything all topsy turvy in your tummy? Fachdolmetschen im Gesundheitsbereich/Health Care Interpreting* (pp. 9–27). Munich: Martin Meidenbauer.

Angelelli, C. V. (2004). *Medical Interpreting and Cross-cultural Communication.* Cambridge: Cambridge University Press. doi: 10.1017/CBO9780511486616

Angelelli, C. V. (2007). Assessing medical interpreters: The language and interpreting testing project. *The Translator, 13*(1), 63–82. https://doi.org/10.1080/1355650 9.2007.10799229

Angelelli, C. V. (2014). Interpreting in the healthcare setting: Access in cross-linguistic communication. In H. Hamilton & S. Chou, S. (Eds), *The Routledge Handbook of Language and Health Communication* (pp. 573–585). London: Routledge.

Azarmina, P., & Wallace, P. (2005). Remote interpretation in medical encounters: A systematic review. *Journal of Telemedicine and Telecare, 11*, 140–145. doi: 10.1258/1357633053688679

Bacigalupe, L. A. (1999). Visual contact in simultaneous interpretation: Results of an experimental study. In A. A. Lugrís & A. F. Ocampo (Eds), *Anovar/Anosar: Estudios de traducción e interpretación* (pp. 123–137). Vigo: University of Vigo.

Baker, D., Hayes, R., & Fortier, J. (1998). Interpreter use and satisfaction with interpersonal aspects of care for Spanish-speaking patients. *Medical Care, 36*(10), 1461–1470. doi: 10.1097/00005650-199810000-00004

Baker, D. W., Parker, R. M., Williams, M. V., Coates, W. C., & Pitkin, K. (1996). Use and effectiveness of interpreters in an emergency department. *Journal of the American Medical Association, 275*(10), 783–788. doi: 10.1001/jama.1996.03530340047028

Baker, M. (2006). *Translation and Conflict: A Narrative Account.* London: Routledge. doi: 10.1001/jama.1996.03530340047028

Balogh, K., & Hertog, E. (2012). AVIDICUS comparative studies – Part II: Traditional, videoconference and remote interpreting in police interviews.

In S. Braun & J. Taylor (Eds), *Videoconference and Remote Interpreting in Criminal Proceedings* (pp. 101–116). Guildford: University of Surrey. <http://www.videoconference-interpreting.net/BraunTaylor2011.html>.

Balogh, K., & Salaets, H. (2018). Videoconferencing in a legal context: A comparative study of simulated and real-life settings. In J. Napier, R. Skinner, & S. Braun (Eds), *Here or There: Research on Interpreting via Video Link* (pp. 264–299). Washington, DC: Gallaudet University Press.

Balzani, M. (1990). Le contact visuel en interprétation simultanée : Résultats d'une expérience (français–italien). In L. Gran & C. Taylor (Eds), *Aspects of Applied and Experimental Research on Conference Interpretation* (pp. 93–100). Udine: Campanotto.

Bao-Rozée, J. (2016). *Using Multimodal Analysis to Investigate the Role of the Interpreter*. Doctoral dissertation. Stirling: University of Stirling.

Baraldi, C., & Gavioli, L. (2007). Dialogue interpreting as intercultural mediation: An analysis in healthcare multicultural settings. In M. Grein & E. Weigand (Eds), *Dialogue and Culture* (pp. 155–176). Amsterdam: John Benjamins. doi: 10.1075/ds.1.12bar

Baraldi, C., & Gavioli, L. (2012). Introduction: Understanding coordination in interpreter-mediated interaction. In C. Baraldi & L. Gavioli (Eds), *Coordinating Participation in Dialogue Interpreting* (pp. 1–22). Amsterdam: John Benjamins. doi: 10.1075/btl.102

Baraldi, C., & Gavioli, L. (2014). Are close renditions the golden standard? Some thoughts on translating accuracy in healthcare interpreter-mediated interaction. *The interpreter and Translator Trainer*, *8*(3), 336–353. doi: 10.1080/1750339X.2014.972029

Barik, H. C. (1971). A description of various types of omissions, additions, and errors of translation encountered in simultaneous interpretation. *Meta, 16*(4), 199–210. doi:10.7202/001972ar

Barik, H. C. (1975). Simultaneous interpretation: Qualitative and linguistic data. *Language and Speech*, *18*(3), 272–297. doi: 10.1177%2F002383097501800310.

Barik, H. C. (1994). A description of various types of omissions, additions and errors of translation encountered in simultaneous interpretation. In S. Lambert & B. Moser-Mercer (Eds), *Bridging the Gap: Empirical Research in Simultaneous Interpretation* (pp. 121–138). Amsterdam: John Benjamins. doi: 10.1075/btl.3.05alt

Bavelas, J., Coates, L., & Johnson, T. (2002). Listener responses as a collaborative process: The role of gaze. *Journal of communication*, *52*(3), 566–580. doi: 10.1111/j.1460-2466.2002.tb02562.x

Besson, C., Graf, D., Hartung, I., Kropfhäusser, B., & Voisard, S. (2005). *The Importance of Nonverbal Communication in Professional Interpretation*.

<http://aiic.net/page /1662/the-importance-of-nonverbal-communication-in-professional-interpretation/lang/1#51>.

Bot, H. (2005). Dialogue Interpreting as a specific case of reported speech. *Interpreting, 7*(2), 237–261. doi: 10.1075/intp.7.2.06bot

Bower, K. (2015). Stress and burnout in Video Relay Service (VRS) interpreting. *Journal of Interpretation, 24*(1), 1–16.

Braun, S. (2003). Kommunikation unter widrigen Umständen? Optimierungsstrategien in zweisprachigen Videokonferenz-Gesprächen. In J. Döring, W. H. Schmitz, & O. A. Schulte (Eds), *Connecting Perspectives. Videokonferenz: Beiträge zu ihrer Erforschung und Anwendung* (pp. 167–185). Aachen: Shaker.

Braun, S. (2004). *Kommunikation unter widrigen Umständen? Fallstudien zu einsprachigen und gedolmetschten Videokonferenzen*. Tübingen: Narr.

Braun, S. (2006). Multimedia communication technologies and their impact on interpreting. In M. Carroll, H. Gerzymisch-Arbogast, & S. Nauert, (Eds), *Proceedings of the Marie Curie Euroconferences MuTra: Audiovisual Translation Scenarios Copenhagen, 1–5 May 2006*. <http://www.euroconferences.info/proceedings/2006_Proceedings/2006_Braun_Sabine.pdf>.

Braun, S. (2007). Interpreting in small-group bilingual videoconferences: Challenges and adaptation processes. *Interpreting, 9*(1), 21–46. doi: 10.1075/intp.9.1.03bra

Braun, S. (2012). Recommendations for the use of video-mediated interpreting in criminal proceedings. In S. Braun & J. L. Taylor (Eds), *Videoconference and Remote Interpreting in Criminal Proceedings* (pp. 265–287). Guildford: University of Surrey. <http://www.videoconference-interpreting.net/BraunTaylor2011.html>.

Braun, S. (2013). Keep your distance? Remote interpreting in legal proceedings: A critical assessment of a growing practice. *Interpreting, 15*(2), 200–228. doi: 10.1075/intp.15.2.03bra

Braun, S. (2015). Remote interpreting. In H. Mikkelson & R. Jourdain (Eds), *The Routledge Handbook of Interpreting* (pp. 352–367). London: Routledge.

Braun, S. (2017). What a micro-analytic investigation of additions and expansions in remote interpreting can tell us about interpreters' participation in a shared virtual space. *Journal of Pragmatics, 107*, 165–177. doi: 10.1016/j.pragma.2016.09.011

Braun, S. (2018). Video-mediated interpreting in legal settings in England: interpreters' perceptions in their sociopolitical context. *Translation and Interpreting Studies, 13*(3), 393–420. doi: 10.1075/tis.00022.bra

Braun, S., & Davitti, E. (2018). Video-mediated interpreting. In A. Amato, N. Spinolo, & M. J. González Rodriguez (Eds), *Handbook of Remote Interpreting. Research Report Shift in Orality Erasmus + Project: Shaping the Interpreters of the Future and of Today* (pp. 103–136). <https://www.shiftinorality.eu/es/resources/2018/05/11/shift-handbook-remote-interpreting>.

Braun, S., Davitti, E., & Dicerto, S. (Eds). (2016). *Handbook of Bilingual Videoconferencing: The Use of Videoconferencing in Proceedings Conducted with the Assistance of an Interpreter.* Guildford: University of Surrey. <http://www.videoconference-interpreting.net/wp-content/uploads/2016/08/AVIDICUS3_Handbook_Bilingual_Video conferencing.pdf>.

Braun, S., & Kohn, K. (2001). Dolmetschen in der Videokonferenz. Kommunikative Kompetenz und Monitoringstrategien. In G. Thome, C. Giehl, & H. Gerzymisch-Arbogast (Eds), *Kultur und Translation: Methodologische Probleme des Kulturtransfers* (pp. 3–32). Tübingen: Narr. EBook: <http://www.translationconcepts.org/pdf/jahrbuch2.pdf>.

Braun, S., & Taylor, J. L. (Eds). (2012a). *Videoconference and Remote Interpreting in Criminal Proceedings.* Guildford: University of Surrey. <http://www.videoconference-interpreting.net/BraunTaylor2011.html>.

Braun, S., & Taylor, J. L. (2012b). AVIDICUS comparative studies – Part I: Traditional interpreting and remote interpreting in police interviews. In S. Braun & J. L. Taylor (Eds), *Videoconference and Remote Interpreting in Criminal Proceedings* (pp. 85–100). Guildford: University of Surrey.

Braun, S., & Taylor, J. (2013). *Developing the Use of Technical Tools in Cross-border Resettlement (DUTT): Videoconference Communication in Cross-border Resettlement.* <https://www.cep-probation.org/wp-content/uploads/2018/10/DUTT-Final-report.pdf>.

Bugel-Shunra, D. (2000). Proofreading translations: A checklist, not a blank check. *ATA Chronicle, 29*(12).

Bühler, H. (1985). Conference interpreting: A multichannel communication phenomenon. *Meta, 30*(1), 49–54. doi: 10.7202/002176ar

Byrne, P. S., & Long, B. E. L. (1984/1976). *Doctors Talking to Patients: A Study of the Verbal Behaviours of Doctors in the Consultation.* Exeter: Royal College of General Practitioners.

Carrasquillo, O., Orav, E. J., Brennan, T. A., & Burstin, H. R. (1999). Impact of language barriers on patient satisfaction in an emergency department. *Journal of General Internal Medicine, 14*(2), 82–87. doi: 10.1046/j.1525-1497.1999.00293.x

Castagnoli, S., & Niemants, N. (2018). Corpora worth creating: A pilot study on telephone interpreting. *InTRAlinea, Special Issue: New Findings in Corpus-based Interpreting Studies.* <http://www.intralinea.org/specials/article/corpora_worth_creating_a_pilot_study_on_telephone_interpreting>.

Chernov, G. V. (2004). *Inference and Anticipation in Simultaneous Interpreting.* Amsterdam: John Benjamins. In P. Mouzourakis (2006). Remote interpreting: A technical perspective on recent experiments. *Interpreting*, *8*(1), 45–66. doi: 10.1075/btl.57

Cirillo, L. (2010). Managing affect in interpreter-mediated institutional talk: Examples from the medical setting. *The Journal of Specialised Translation*, *14*, 55–79. <https://www.jostrans.org/issue14/art_cirillo.pdf>.

Clancy, P. M., Thompson, S. A., & Suzuki, R. (1996). The conversational use of reactive tokens in English, Japanese, and Mandarin. *Journal of Pragmatics*, *26*(3), 355–387. doi: 10.1016/0378-2166(95)00036-4

Cokely, D. (1992). *Interpretation: A Sociolinguistic Model*. Burtonsville, MD: Linstok.

Corey, J., Garruba, M., & Melder, A. (2017). Patient satisfaction of telephone or video interpreter services compared with in-person services: A systematic review. *Australian Health Review*, *42*(2), 168–177. doi: 10.1071/AH16195

Crossman, K. L., Wiener, E., Roosevelt, G., Bajaj, L., & Hampers, L. C. (2010). Interpreters: Telephonic, in-person interpretation and bilingual providers. *Pediatrics*, *125*(3), 631–638. doi: 10.1542/peds.2009-0769

Cunningham, H., Cushman, L. F., Akuete-Penn, C., & Meyer, D. D. (2008). Satisfaction with telephonic interpreters in pediatric care. *Journal of the National Medical Association*, *100*(4), 429–434. doi: 10.1016/S0027-9684(15)31277-3

Davidson, B. (2002). A model for the construction of conversational common ground in interpreted discourse. *Journal of Pragmatics*, *34*, 1273–1300.

Davitti, E. (2012). *Dialogue Interpreting as Intercultural Mediation Integrating Talk and Gaze in the Analysis of Mediated Parent-teacher Meetings*. PhD thesis. Manchester: University of Manchester. <https://www.escholar.manchester.ac.uk/api/datastream?publicationPid=uk-ac-man-scw:162289&datastreamId=FULL-TEXT.PDF>.

Davitti, E. (2013). Dialogue interpreting as intercultural mediation: Interpreters' use of upgrading moves in parent-teacher meetings. *Interpreting*, *15*(2), 168–199. doi: 10.1075/intp. 15.2.02dav

Davitti, E. (2018). Methodological explorations of interpreter-mediated interaction: Novel insights from multimodal analysis. *Qualitative Research*, *19*(1), 7–29. doi: 10.1177%2F1468794118761492

Davitti, E., & Braun, S. (2018). Challenges and solutions. In A. Amato, N. Spinolo, & M. J. González Rodríguez (Eds), *Handbook of Remote Interpreting: Research Report Shift in Orality Erasmus + Project: Shaping the Interpreters of the Future and of Today* (pp. 119–135). <https://www.shiftinorality.eu/es/resources/2018/05/11/shift-handbook-remote-interpreting>.

Davitti, E., & Braun, S. (2020). Analysing interactional phenomena in video remote interpreting in collaborative settings: Implications for interpreter education.

The Interpreter and Translator Trainer, 14 (3), 279 -302. https://doi.org/10.108 0/1750399X.2020.1800364

Davitti, E., & Pasquandrea, S. (2017). Embodied participation: What multimodal analysis can tell us about interpreter-mediated encounters in pedagogical settings. *Journal of Pragmatics, 107*, 105–128. doi: 10.1016/j.pragma.2016.04.008

De Bontridder, R., & De Groote, R. (2014). *Handboek: Basisopleiding sociaal tolken.* Brussel: Agentschap Integratie en Inburgering. <https://ec.europa.eu/educat ion/knowledge-centre-interpretation/sites/default/files/handboeksociaalto lken_20171201_0.pdf>.

Eggins, S. (1994). *An Introduction to Systemic Functional Linguistics.* London: Pinter.

Ellis, S. R. (2004). Videoconferencing in refugee hearings. *Ellis Report to the Immigration and Refugee Board Audit and Evaluation Committee.* <https:// irb-cisr.gc.ca/en/transparency/reviews-audit-evaluations/Pages/Video.aspx>.

Englund Dimitrova, B. (1997). Degree of interpreter responsibility in the interaction process in community interpreting. In S. E. Carr (Ed), *The Critical Link: Interpreters in the Community* (pp. 147–164). Amsterdam: Benjamins. doi:10.1075/btl.19.17eng

Englund Dimitrova, B., & Tiselius, E. (2016). Cognitive aspects of community interpreting. Toward a process model. In R. Muñoz Martín (Ed.), *Reembedding Translation Process Research* (pp. 195–214). Amsterdam: John Benjamins. doi: 10.1075/btl.128.10eng

Esteban Causo, J. (2012). Conference interpreting with information and communication technologies: Experiences from the European Commission DG Interpretation. In S. Braun & J. L. Taylor (Eds), *Videoconference and Remote Interpreting in Criminal Proceedings* (pp. 199–203). Guildford: University of Surrey. <http://www.videoconference-interpreting.net/BraunTaylor2011. html>.

Fagan, M. J., Diaz, J. A., Reinert, S. E., Sciamanna, C. N., & Fagan, D. M. (2003). Impact of interpretation method on clinic visit length. *Journal of General Internal Medicine, 18*, 634–638. doi: 10.1046/j.1525-1497.2003.20701.x

Fantinuoli, C. (2018). Interpreting and technology: The upcoming technological turn. In C. Fantinuoli (Ed.), *Interpreting and Technology* (pp. 1–12). Berlin: Language Science Press.

Fantinuoli, C. (2022). Conference interpreting and new technologies. In M. Albl-Mikasa & E. Tiselius (Eds), *The Routledge Handbook of Conference Interpreting* (pp. 508–523). London: Routledge. doi: 10.4324/9780429297878-44

Farlex. (2012). *The Free Dictionary by Farlex – Farlex Partner Medical Dictionary.* <https://medical-dictionary.thefreedictionary.com/ rapport>.

Fernández-Pérez, M. (2017). Interaction management skills in telephone interpreting. *Revista canaria de estudios ingleses*, *75*, 103–117.

Flores, G., Abreu, M., Barone, C. P., Bachur, R., & Lin, H. (2012). Errors of medical interpretation and their potential clinical consequences: A comparison of professional versus ad hoc versus no interpreters. *Annals of Emergency Medicine*, *60*(5), 545–553. doi: 10.1016/j.annemergmed.2012.01.025

Flores, G., Abreu, M., Olivar, M. A., & Kastner, B. (1998). Access barriers to health care for Latino children. *Archives of Pediatrics and Adolescent Medicine*, *152*(11), 1119–1125. doi: 10.1001/archpedi.152.11.1119

Flores, G., Laws, M. B., Mayo, S. J., Zuckerman, B., Abreu, M., Medina, L., & Hardt, E. J. (2003). Errors in medical interpretation and their potential clinical consequences in pediatric encounters. *Pediatrics*, *111*(1), 6–14. doi: 10.1542/peds.111.1.6

Fowler, Y. (2007). Interpreting into the ether: Interpreting for prison/court video link hearings. *Proceedings of the Critical Link 5 Conference, Sydney*. <http://criticallink.org/cli-5/>.

Gallez, E. (2021). Un format horizontal pour transcrire et analyser les interactions triadiques interprétées. *The Interpreter's Newsletter*, *26*, 55–75. <http://hdl.handle.net/10077/33262>.

Gany, F., Kapelusznik, L., Prakash, K., Gonzalez, J., Orta, L. Y., & Tseng, C. H. (2007a). The impact of medical interpretation method on time and errors. *Journal of General Internal Medicine*, *22*(2), 319–323. doi: 10.1007/s11606-007-0361-7

Gany, F., Lang, J., Shapiro, E., Abramson, D., Motola, I., Shield, D. C., & Changrani, J. (2007b). Patient satisfaction with different interpreting methods: A randomized controlled trial. *Journal of General Internal Medicine*, *22*(2), 312–318. doi: 10.1007/s11606-007-0360-8

Garcia, E., Roy, L., Okada, P., Perkins, S., & Wiebe, R. (2004). A comparison of the influence of hospital-trained, ad hoc, and telephone interpreters on perceived satisfaction of limited English-proficient parents presenting to a pediatric emergency department. *Pediatric Emergency Care*, *20*(6), 373–378. doi: 10.1097/01.pec.0000133611.42699.08

Gardner, R. (2001). *When Listeners Talk: Response Tokens and Listener Stance*. Amsterdam: John Benjamins. <https://doi.org/10.1075/pbns.92>.

Gavioli, L. (2012). Minimal responses in interpreter-mediated talk. In C. Baraldi & L. Gavioli (Eds), *Coordinating Participation in Dialogue Interpreting* (pp. 201–228). Amsterdam: John Benjamins. doi: 10.1075/btl.102

Gerver, D. (1975). A psychological approach to simultaneous interpreting. *Meta*, *20*(2), 119–128. https://doi.org/10.7202/002885ar

Gerwing, J., & Li, S. (2019). Body-oriented gestures as a practioner's window into interpreted communication. *Social Science and Medicine*, *233*, 171–180. doi: 10.1016/j.socscimed.2019.05.040

Gile, D. (1992). Basic theoretical components for interpreter and translator training. In C. Dollerup & A. Loddegaard (Eds), *Teaching Translation and Interpreting: Training, Talent and Experience. Papers from the First Language International Conference*. Amsterdam: John Benjamins. doi: 10.1075/z.56

Gile, D. (1995). *Basic Concepts and Models for Interpreter and Translator Training*. Amsterdam: John Benjamins. doi: 10.1075/btl.8(1st)

Goffman, E. (1981). *Forms of Talk*. Philadelphia: Pennsylvania Press.

González Rodríguez, M. J. (2018). Basic requirements and prerequisites for successful communication with remote interpreting. In A. Amato, N. Spinolo, & M. J. González Rodríguez (Eds), *Handbook of Remote Interpreting: Research Report Shift in Orality Erasmus + Project: Shaping the Interpreters of the Future and of Today* (pp. 138–141). <https://www.shiftinorality.eu/es/resources/2018/05/11/shift-handbook-remote-interpreting>.

González Rodríguez, M. J., & Spinolo, N. (2017). Telephonic dialogue interpreting. In N. Niemants & L. Cirillo (Eds), *Teaching Dialogue Interpreting* (pp. 242–257). Amsterdam: John Benjamins. doi: 10.1075/btl.138.12gon

Goodwin, C. (1979). The interactive construction of a sentence in natural conversation. In G. Psathas (Ed.), *Everyday Language: Studies in Ethnomethodology* (pp. 97–121). New York: Irvington.

Goodwin, C. (1981). *Conversational Organization Interaction between Speakers and Hearers*. New York: Academic Press.

Goodwin, M. H., & Goodwin, C. (1986). Gesture and coparticipation in the activity of searching for a word. *Semiotica*, *62*, 51–75.

Grbić, N. (2015). Quality. In F. Pöchhacker, N. Grbić, P. Mead, & R. Setton (Eds), *Routledge Encyclopedia of Interpreting Studies* (pp. 333–337). London: Routledge. doi: 10.4324/9781315678467

Gumperz, J. J. (1982). *Discourse Strategies*. Cambridge: Cambridge University Press. doi: 10.1017/CBO9780511611834

Gumperz, J. J. (2005). Interactional sociolinguistics: A personal perspective. In D. Schiffrin, D. Tannen, & H. Hamilton (Eds), *The Handbook of Discourse Analysis* (pp. 215–218). Cambridge, MA: Blackwell. doi: 10.1002/9780470753460.ch12

Hale, S. (2004). *The Discourse of Court Interpreting: Discourse Practices of the Law, the Witness and the Interpreter*. Amsterdam: John Benjamins. doi: 10.1075/btl.52

Hale, S. (2007). *Community Interpreting*. Basingstoke: Palgrave Macmillan.

Hale, S., & Napier, J. (2013). *Research Methods in Interpreting Studies: A Practical Resource*. London: Bloomsbury.

Hampers, L. C., Cha, S., Gutglass, D. J., Binns, H. J., & Krug, S. E. (1999). Language barriers and resource utilization in a pediatric emergency department. *Pediatrics, 103*(6–1), 1253–1256. doi: 10.1542/peds.103.6.1253

Hampers, L., & McNulty, J. (2002). Professional interpreters and bilingual physicians in a pediatric emergency department: Effect on resource utilization. *Archives of Pediatrics and Adolescent Medecine, 156*(11), 1108–1113. doi: 10.1001/archpedi.156.11.1108

Hansen, J. P. B. (2020). Invisible participants in a visual ecology: Visual space as a resource for organizing video-mediated interpreting in hospital encounters. *Social Interaction. Video-based Studies of Human Sociality, 3*(3), 1–25. doi: 10.7146/si.v3i3.122609

Hansen, J. P. B., & Svennevig, J. (2021). Creating space for interpreting within extended turns at talk. *Journal of Pragmatics, 182*, 144–162. doi: 10.1016/j.pragma.2021.06.009

Harmsen, J. A. M., Bernsen, R. M. D., Meeuwesen, L., Pinto, D., & Bruijnzeels, M. A. (2005). Assessment of mutual understanding of physician patient encounters: Development and validation of a mutual understanding scale (MUS) in a multicultural general practice setting. *Patient Education and Counseling, 59*, 171–181.

Hatim, B., & Mason, I. (1990). *Discourse and the Translator*. London: Longman.

Havelka, I. (2018). *Videodolmetschen im Gesundheitswesen: Dolmetschwissenschaftliche Untersuchung eines österreichisches Pilotprojektes*. Berlin: Frank & Timme.

Heath, C. (1992). The delivery and reception of diagnosis in the general-practice consultation. In P. Drew & J. Heritage (Eds), *Talk at Work: Interaction in Institutional Settings* (pp. 235–267). Cambridge: Cambridge University Press.

Heath, C. (1986/2004). *Body Movement and Speech in Medical Interaction*. Cambridge: Cambridge University Press.

Herbert, J. (1952). *The Interpreter's Handbook: How to Become a Conference Interpreter*. Geneva: Georg.

Heritage, J., & Maynard, D. W. (2006). *Communication in Medical Care: Interaction between Primary Care Physicians and Patients*. Cambridge: Cambridge University Press. doi: 10.1017/CBO9780511607172

Herring, R. H. (2019). "A lot to think about": Online monitoring in dialogue interpreting. *Translation, Cognition & Behavior, 2*(2), 283–304.

Hlavac, J. (2013). Should interpreters be trained and tested in telephone and video-link interpreting?: Responses from practitioners and examiners. *International Journal of Interpreter Education, 5*(1), 34–50. doi: 10.12807/ti.105201.2013.a02

Hornberger, J., Gibson, C. D., Wood, W., Dequeldre, C., Corso, I., Palla, B., & Bloch, D. A. (1996). Eliminating language barriers for non-English-speaking patients. *Medical Care, 34*(8), 845–856. doi: 10.1097/00005650-199608000-00011

Hsieh, E. (2007). Interpreters as co-diagnosticians: Overlapping roles and services between providers and interpreters. *Social Science & Medicine, 64*, 924–937. doi: 10.1016/j.socscimed.2006.10.015

Hsieh, E. (2016). *Bilingual Health Communication: Working with Interpreters in Cross-cultural Care*. London: Routledge.

Hsieh, E. (2017). The model of bilingual health communication: Theorizing interpreter-mediated medical encounters. In E. A. Jacobs & L. C. Diamond (Eds), *Providing Health Care in the Context of Language Barriers: International Perspectives* (pp. 35–55). Bristol: Multilingual Matters. doi: 10.21832/9781783097777-005

Hsieh, E., & Hong, S. J. (2010). Interpreters in healthcare – Not all desired: Providers' views on interpreters' emotional support for patients. *Patient Education and Counseling, 81*, 192–197. doi: 10.1016/j.pec.2010.04.004

Hsieh, E., & Kramer, E. M. (2021). *Rethinking Culture in Health Communication: Social Interaction as Intercultural Encounters*. Hoboken, NJ: John Wiley & Sons.

Iglesias-Fernández, E. (2010). Verbal and nonverbal concomitants of rapport in health care encounters: Implications for interpreters. *The Journal of Specialized Translation, 14*, 216–227.

Iglesias-Fernández, E., & Russo, M. (2020). A multidisciplinary theoretical and methodological framework for the study of telephone interpreting. *The Interpreter and Translator Trainer, 14*(3), 240–258. doi: 10.1080/1750399X.2020.1800363

ITU/ETI/Swisscom. (1999). Background paper to interim report on remote interpretation. International Telecommunications Union, Ecole de traduction et d'interprétation, Swisscom. Report published for IAMLAPD 1999, Rome, WFP. Geneva : ITU/ETI.

Jefferson, G. (2004). Glossary of transcript symbols with an introduction. In G. H. Lerner (Ed.), *Conversation Analysis: Studies from the First Generation*. Amsterdam: John Benjamins. doi: 10.1075/pbns.125.02jef

Jewitt, C. (Ed.). (2009). *The Routledge Handbook of Multimodal Analysis*. London: Routledge.

Jones, D., Gill, P., Harrison, R., Meakin, R., & Wallace, P. (2003). An exploratory study of language interpretation services provided by videoconferencing. *Journal of Telemedicine and Telecare, 9*, 51–56. doi: 10.1258/135763303321159701

Kaufert, J. M., & Koolidge, W. W. (1984). Role conflict among "culture brokers": The experience of native Canadian medical interpreters. *Social Science & Medicine, 18*(3), 283–286. doi: 10.1016/0277-9536(84)90092-3

Ko, L. (2006). The need for long-term empirical studies in remote interpreting research: A case study of telephone interpreting. *Linguistica Antverpiensia – Themes in Translation Studies, 5*, 325–338.

Kelly, N. (2008). *Telephone Interpreting: A Comprehensive Guide to the Profession*. Victoria, BC: Trafford Publishing.

Kendon, A. (1967). Some functions of gaze direction in social interaction. *Acta Psychologica, 26*, 22–63. doi:10.1016/0001-6918(67)90005-4

Klebnikov, G. (1979). Remote interpretation experiment – United Nations Headquarters, 5 & 7 September. *AIIC Bulletin, 6*(2), 169–175.

Koller, M., & Pöchhacker, F. (2018). The work and skills … a profile of first-generation video remote interpreters. In J. Napier, R. Skinner, & S. Braun (Eds), *Here or There: Research on Interpreting via Video Link* (pp. 89–110). Washington, DC: Gallaudet University Press.

Korak, C. (2010). *Remote Interpreting via Skype. Anwendungsmöglichkeiten von VoIP Software im Bereich Community Interpreting – Communicate Everywhere?* Berlin: Frank & Timme.

Kress, G., & Van Leeuwen, T. (2001). *Multimodal Discourse: The Modes and Media of Contemporary Communication*. Oxford: Oxford University Press.

Krystallidou, D. (2014). Gaze and body orientation as an apparatus for patient inclusion into/exclusion from a patient-centred framework of communication. *The Interpreter and Translator Trainer, 8*(3), 399–417. doi: 10.1080/1750399X.2014.972033

Krystallidou, D. (2016). Investigating the interpreter's role(s). The A.R.T. framework. *Interpreting, 18*(2), 172–197. doi: 10.1075/intp.18.2.02kry

Krystallidou, D., Remael, A., de Boe, E., Hendrickx, K., Tzakitzidis, G., Van de Geuchte, S., & Pype, P. (2018). Investigating empathy in interpreter-mediated simulated consultations: An explorative study. *Patient Education and Counseling, 101*(1), 33–42. doi: 10.1016/j.pec.2017.07.022

Kuo, D., & Fagan, M. J. (1999). Satisfaction with methods of Spanish interpretation in an ambulatory care clinic. *Journal of General Internal Medicine, 14*, 547–50. doi: 10.1046/j.1525-1497.1999.07258.x

Kurz, I. (1996). Interpreting: Sound vs. sound and picture. *The Jerome Quarterly, 12*(1), 5–14.

Kurz, I. (1999). Remote conference interpreting: Assessing the technology. H. N. Helge (coord.) "Quality issues in remote interpreting". A.A. Lugris & A.F. Ocampo (Eds). *Anovar/anosar Estudios de Tranduccion e Interpretación*, 1, Servicio de Publicacion da Universidade de Vigo, 114–116.

Kurz, I. (2000). Tagungsort Genf/Nairobi/Wien: Zu einigen Aspekten des Teledolmetschens. In M. Kadric, K. Kaindl, & F. Pöchhacker (Eds), *Festschrift für Mary Snell-Hornby zum 60. Geburtstag* (pp. 291–302). Tübingen: Stauffenburg.

Kussmaul, P. (1995). *Training the Translator*. Amsterdam: John Benjamins. doi: 10.1075/btl.10

Lee, J. (2007). Telephone interpreting – Seen from the interpreter's perspective. *Interpreting, 9*(2), 231–252. doi: 10.1075/intp.9.2.05lee

Lee, L., Batal, H. A., Maselli, J. H., & Kutner, J. S. (2002). Effect of Spanish interpretation method on patient satisfaction in an urban walk-in clinic. *Journal of General Internal Medicine, 17*(8), 641–645. doi: 10.1046/j.1525-1497.2002.10742.x

Licoppe, C., & Vernier, M. (2013). Interpreting, video communication and the sequential reshaping of institutional talk in the bilingual and distributed courtroom. *International Journal of Speech, Language and the Law, 20,* 247–275. doi: 10.1558/ijsll.v20i2.247

Licoppe, C., & Veyrier, C. (2017). How to show the interpreter on screen? The normative organization of visual ecologies in multilingual courtrooms with video links. *Journal of Pragmatics, 107,* 147–164. doi: 10.1016/j.pragma.2016.09.012

Llewllyn-Jones, P., & Lee, R. (2014). *Redefining the Role of the Community Interpreter: The Concept of Role-space.* Lincoln: SLI Press.

Locatis, C., Williamson, D., Gould-Kabler, C., Zone-Smith, L., Detzler, I., Roberson, J., Maisiak, R., & Ackerman, M. (2010). Comparing in-person, video, and telephonic medical interpretation. *Journal of General Internal Medicine, 25*(4), 345–350. doi: 10.1007/s11606-009-1236-x

Locatis, C., Williamson, D., Sterrett, J., Detzler, I., & Ackerman, M. (2011). Video medical interpretation over 3G cellular networks: A feasibility study. *Telemedicine and e-Health, 17*(10), 809–813. doi: 10.1089/tmj.2011.0084

Major, G., & Napier, J. (2012). Interpreting and knowledge mediation in the healthcare setting: What do we really mean by "accuracy"? *Linguistica Antverpiensia – New Series: Themes in Translation Studies, 11,* 207–225.

Masland, M. C., Lou, C., & Snowden, L. (2010). Use of communication technologies to cost-effectively increase the availability of interpretation services in healthcare settings. *Telemedicine and e-Health, 16*(6), 739–745. doi: 10.1089/tmj.2009.0186

Mason, I. (1999). Introduction. *The Translator, 5*(2), 147–160. doi:10.1080/13556509.1999.10799038

Mason, I. (2000). Models and methods in dialogue interpreting research. In M. Olohan (Ed.), *Intercultural Fault Lines. Research Models in Translation Studies I: Textual and Cognitive Aspects* (pp. 215–232). Manchester: St Jerome Publishing. doi: 10.4324/9781315759951-14

Mason, I. (2001). *Triadic Exchanges. Studies in Dialogue Interpreting.* Manchester: St Jerome.

Mason, I. (2012). Gaze, positioning and identity in interpreter-mediated dialogues. In C. Baraldi & L. Gavioli (Eds), *Coordinating Participation in Dialogue*

Interpreting (pp. 177–199). Amsterdam: John Benjamins. doi: 10.1075/btl.102.08mas

Mason, M., & Rock, F. (2019). *The Discourse of Police Interviews.* Chicago: University of Chicago Press. doi: 10.7208/chicago/9780226647821.001.0001

Maxwell, J. A. (2013). *Qualitative Research Design: An Interactive Approach.* Thousand Oaks, CA: Sage Publications.

MacCulloch, C. E., & Searle, S. R. (2001). *Generalized, Linear, and Mixed Models.* Hoboken, NJ: Wiley. doi: 10.1002/0471722073

Meeuwesen, L., Twilt, S., Ten Thije, J. D., & Harmsen, H. (2010). "Ne diyor?" (What does she say?): Informal interpreting in general practice. *Patient Education and Counseling, 81,* 198–203. doi: 10.1016/j.pec.2009.10.005

Mercer, S. W., & Reynolds, W. J. (2002). Empathy and quality of care. *The British Journal of General Practice: The Journal of the Royal College of General Practitioners, 52*(Suppl), S9–S12.

Merlini, R., & Favaron, R. (2007). Examining the "voice of interpreting" in speech pathology. In M. Schlesinger & F. Pöchhacker (Eds), *Healthcare Interpreting* (pp. 101–139). Amsterdam: John Benjamins. doi: 10.1075bct.9.08mer

Metzger, M. (1999). *Sign Language Interpreting: Deconstructing the Myth of Neutrality.* Washington, DC: Gallaudet University Press.

Mishler, E. G. (1984). *The discourse of Medicine: Dialectics of Medical Interviews.* Norwood, NJ: Ablex.

Mondada, L. (2007). Multimodal resources for turn-taking: Pointing and the emergence of possible next speakers. *Discourse Studies, 9*(2), 195–226.

Mondada, L. (2011). Understanding as an embodied, situated and sequential achievement in interaction. *Journal of Pragmatics, 43,* 542–552.

Mondada, L. (2016). Challenges of multimodality: Language and the body in social interaction. *Journal of Sociolinguistics, 20*(3), 336–366. doi: 10.1111/josl.1_12177

Monteoliva-García, E. (2020). The collaborative and selective nature of interpreting in police interviews with stand-by interpreting. *Interpreting, 22*(2), 262–287. doi:10.1075/intp.00046.mon

Morse, J., Anderson, G., Bottorff, J. L., Yonge, O., O'Brien, B., Solberg, S. M., & McIlveen, K. H. (1992). Exploring empathy: A conceptual fit for nursing practice? *The Journal of Nursing Scholarship, 24*(4), 273–280. doi: 10.1111/j.1547-5069.1992.tb00733.x

Moser-Mercer, B. (2003). Remote interpreting: Assessment of human factors and performance parameters. *Communicate*! <http://aiic.net/ViewPage.cfm?page_id=1125>.

Moser-Mercer, B. (2005a). Remote interpreting: Issues of multi-sensory integration in a multilingual task. *Meta, 50*(2), 727–738. doi: 10.7202/011014ar

Moser-Mercer, B. (2005b). Remote interpreting: The crucial role of presence. *Bulletin suisse de linguistique appliqué, 81*, 73–97.
Mouzourakis, P. (1996). Videoconferencing: Techniques and challenges. *Interpreting, 1*(1), 21–38. doi: 10.1075/intp.1.1.03mou
Mouzourakis, P. (2000). *Interpretation Booths for the Third Millennium.* <http://aiic.net/page/131/interpretation-booths-for-the-third-millennium>.
Mouzourakis, P. (2003). That feeling of being there: Vision and presence in remote interpreting. *Communicate!* <http://www.aiic.net/ViewPage.cfm/article911.htm>.
Mouzourakis, P. (2006). Remote interpreting: A technical perspective on recent experiments. *Interpreting, 8*(1), 45–66. doi: 10.1075/intp.8.1.04mou
Muñoz-Martín, M. R. (2014). Situating translation expertise: A review with a sketch of a construct. In J. Schwieter & A. Ferreira (Eds), *The Development of Translation Competence: Theories and Methodologies from Psycholinguistics and Cognitive Science* (pp. 2–54). Cambridge: Cambridge Scholars Publishing.
Napier, J. (2004). Interpreting omissions: A new perspective. *Interpreting, 6*(2), 117–142. doi: 10.1075/intp.6.2.02nap
Napier, J., & Leneham, M. (2011). "It was difficult to manage the communication": Testing the feasibility of video remote signed language interpreting in court. *Journal of Interpretation, 21*(1), Article 5. <http://digitalcommons.unf.edu/joi/vol21/iss1/5>.
Napier, J., Skinner, R., & Turner, G. H. (2018). Enabling political participation through remote interpreting: A case study. In J. Napier, R. Skinner, & S. Braun (Eds), *Here or There: Research on Interpreting via Video Link* (pp. 230–236). Washington, DC: Gallaudet University Press.
Nápoles, A. M, Santoyo-Olsson, J., Karliner, L.S. O'Brien, H., Gregorich, S. E., Pérez-Stable, E. J. (2010). Clinician ratings of interpreter mediated visits in underserved primary care settings with ad hoc, in-person professional, and video conferencing modes. *Journal of Healthcare for the Poor und Underserved, 21*(1), 301–317. doi:10.1353/hpu.0.0269
Ng, E. N. S., & Crezee, I. (2020). *Interpreting in Legal and Healthcare Settings: Perspectives on Research and Training.* Amsterdam: John Benjamins. doi: 10.1075/btl.151
Niska, H. (1999). Quality issues in remote interpreting. In A. Álvarez Lugris & A. Fernández Ocampo (Eds), *Anovar/Anosar estudios de traduccion e interpretaccion* (pp. 109–121). Vigo: University of Vigo.
Norris, S. (2004). *Analyzing Multimodal Interaction: A Methodological Framework.* London: Routledge. doi: 10.4324/9780203379493

Norris, S. (2009). Tempo, Auftakt, levels of actions, and practice: Rhythm in ordinary interactions. *Journal of Applied Linguistics*, *6*(3), 333–355. doi: 10.1558/japl.v6i3.333

O'Connaill, B., Whittaker, S., & Wilbur, S. (1997). Conversation over videoconferences: An evaluation of the spoken aspects of video-mediated communication. *Human-Computer Interaction*, *7*, 374–374.

O'Hagan, M. (1996). *The Coming Industry of Teletranslation*. Clevedon: Multilingual Matters.

O'Hagan, M., & Ashworth, D. (2002). *Translation-mediated Communication in a Digital World*. Clevedon: Multilingual Matters. doi: 10.21832/9781853595820

Oléron, P., & Nanpon, H. (1965). Recherches sur la traduction simultanée [Studies of simultaneous translation]. *Journal de Psychologie Normale et Pathologique*, *62*(1), 73–94.

Oloff, F. (2013). Embodied withdrawal after overlap resolution. *Journal of Pragmatics*, *46*(1), 139–156. doi: 10.1016/j.pragma.2012.07.005

Olson, J., Olson, G., & Meader, D. (1997). Face-to-face group work compared to remote group work. In K. Finn, A. Sellen, & S. Wilbur (Eds), *Video-mediated Communication* (pp. 323–347). Mahwah, NJ: Lawrence Erlbaum.

O'Malley, C., Langton, S., Anderson, A., Doherty-Sneddon, G., & Bruce, V. (1996). Comparison of face-to-face and video-mediated communication. *Interacting-with-Computers*, *8*(2), 177–192. doi: 10.1016/0953-5438(96)01027-2

Oviatt, S., & Cohen, P. (1992). Spoken language in interpreted telephone dialogues. *Computer Speech and Language*, *6*, 277–302. doi: 10.1016/0885-2308(92)90021-U

Ozolins, U. (2011). Telephone interpreting: Understanding practice and identifying research needs. *Translation & Interpreting*, *3*(1).

Paras, M., Leyva, O., Berthold, T., & Otake, R. (2002). *Videoconferencing Medical Interpretation: The Results of Clinical Trials*. Oakland, CA: Health Access Foundation.

Pittarello, S. (2012). Medical terminology and interactional organisation in interpreter-mediated medical encounters. *Linguistica Antverpiensia, New Series – Themes in Translation Studies*, *11*, 113–131.

Pasquandrea, S. (2011). Managing multiple actions through multimodality: Doctor's involvement in interpreter-mediated interactions. *Language in Society*, *40*, 455–481. doi:10.1017/S0047404511000479

Pöchhacker, F. (2001). Quality assessment in conference and community interpreting. *Meta*, *46*(2), 410–425. doi: 10.7202/003847ar

Pöchhacker, F. (2016/2004). *Introducing Interpreting Studies*. London: Routledge. doi: 10.4324//9781315649573/9780203504802

Pöchhacker, F. (2006). Research and methodology in healthcare interpreting. *Linguistica Antverpiensia, New Series – Themes in Translation Studies, 5,* 135–159.
Pöchhacker, F. (2014). Remote possibilities: Training simultaneous video interpreting for Austrian Hospitals. In B. Nicodemus & M. Metzger (Eds), *Investigations in Healthcare Interpreting* (pp. 302–326). Washington, DC: Gallaudet University Press.
Pöchhacker, F., & Schlesinger, M. (2005). Introduction: Discourse based research on healthcare interpreting. *Interpreting, 7*(2), 157–165. doi: 10.1075/intp.7.2.01poc
Pöchhacker, F., & Shlesinger, M. (Eds) (2002). *The Interpreting Studies Reader.* London: Routledge.
Pointon, T., Ozolins, U., & Doucouliagos, C. (1998). *TIS in Europe 1976–2001: Determining the Origins, Size, Nature & Outlook of Telephone Interpreting Services in Europe.* London: The Pointon Partnership/Deakin University.
Price Leemann, E., Pérez-Stabel, E. J., Nickleach, D., López, M., & Karliner, L. S. (2012). Interpreter perspectives of in-person, telephonic, and videoconferencing medical interpretation in clinical encounters. *Patient Education and Counseling, 87*(2), 226–232. doi: 10.1016/j.pec.2011.08.006
Reynolds, W. J., & Scott, B. (1999). Empathy: A crucial component of the helping relationship. *Journal of Psychiatric and Mental Health Nursing, 6,* 363–370. doi: 10.1046/j.1365-2850.1999.00228.x.
Rosenberg, B. A. (2007). A data driven analysis of telephone interpreting. In C. Wadensjö, B. Englund Dimitrova, & A. L. Nilsson (Eds), *The Critical Link 4: Professionalisation of Interpreting in the Community* (pp. 65–76). Amsterdam: John Benjamins. doi: 10.1075/btl.70. 09ros
Rossano, F., Brown, P., & Levinson, S. C. (2009). Gaze, questioning and culture. In J. Sidnell (Ed.), *Conversation Analysis: Comparative Perspectives* (pp. 187–249). Cambridge: Cambridge University Press. doi: 10.1017/CBO9780511635670.008
Roy, C. (2000). *Interpreting as a Discourse Process.* New York: Oxford University Press.
Rozinei, I., & Shlesinger, M. (2010). Much ado about something remote: Stress and performance in remote interpreting. *Interpreting, 12*(2), 214–247. doi: 10.1075/intp.12.2.05roz
Sacks, H., Shegloff, E. A., & Jefferson, G. (1974). A simplest systematics for the organization of turn-taking in conversation. *Language, 50,* 696–736. doi: 10.1353/lan.1974.0010
Saint-Louis, L., Friedman, E., Chiasson, E., Quessa, A., & Novaes, F. (2003). *Testing New Technologies in Medical Interpreting.* Somerville, MA: Cambridge Health Alliance. <https://icommunityhealth.org/wp-content/uploads/2003/06/Testing-New-Technologies-in-Medical-Interpreting.pdf>.

Schegloff, Emanuel A. (1972). Notes on a conversational practice: Formulating place. In D. Sudnow (Ed), *Studies in social interaction* (pp. 75–119). New York: Free Press.

Schegloff, E. A. (1982). Discourse as an interactional achievement: Some uses of "Uh Huh" and other things that come between sentences. In D. Tannen (Ed.), *Georgetown University Round Table on Languages and Linguistics, Analyzing Discourse: Text and Talk* (pp. 71–93). Washington, DC: Georgetown University Press.

Schegloff, E. (2000). Overlapping talk and the organization of turn-taking for conversation. *Language in Society*, *29*(1), 1–63. <https://doi.org/10.1017/S0047404500001019>.

Schegloff, E. A. (1996). Turn organization: One intersection of grammar and interaction. In E. Ochs, E. A. Schegloff, & S. A. Thompson (Eds), *Interaction and Grammar* (pp. 52–133). Cambridge: Cambridge University Press. doi: 10.1017/CBO9780511620874.002

Schegloff, E. A., Jefferson, G., & Sacks, H. (1977). The preference for self-correction in the organization of repair in conversation. *Language*, *53*(2), 361–382. doi: 10.1353/lan.1977.0041

Schiffrin, D. (1994). *Approaches to Discourse*. Cambridge, MA: Blackwell.

Schouten, B. C., Cox, A., Duran, G., Kerremans, K., Köseoğlu-Banning, L., Lahdidioui, A., Van den Muijsenbergh, M., Schinkel, S. Sungur, H., Suurmond, J., Zendedel, R., & Krystallidou, D. (2020). Mitigating language and cultural barriers in healthcare communication: Toward a holistic approach. *Patient Education and Counseling*, *103*(12), 2604–2608. doi: 10.1016/j.pec.2020.05.001

Seeber, K. G., & Fox, B. (2022). Distance conference interpreting. In M. Albl-Mikasa & E. Tiselius (Eds), *The Routledge Handbook of Conference Interpreting* (pp. 491–508). London: Routledge. doi: 10.4324/9780429297878-43

Sellen, A. (1995). Remote conversations: The effects of mediating talk with technology. *Human-Computer Interaction*, *10*(4), 401–444. doi: 10.1207/s15327051hci1004_2

Sellen, A., & Harper, R. (1997). Video in support of organisational talk. In K. Finn, A. Sellen, & S. Wilbur (Eds), *Video-mediated Communication* (pp. 225–243). Mahwah, NJ: Lawrence Erlbaum.

Setton, R. (1999). *Simultaneous Interpretation. A Cognitive-pragmatic Analysis*. Amsterdam: John Benjamins. doi: 10.1075/btl.28

Shlesinger, M. (2007). Quality in simultaneous interpreting. In Y. Gambier, D. Gile, & C. Taylor (Eds), *Conference Interpreting: Current Trends in Research* (pp. 123–131). Amsterdam: John Benjamins. doi: 10.1075/btl.23.08shl

Shlesinger, M. (2009). Crossing the divide: What researchers and practitioners can learn from one another. *Translation & Interpreting*, *1*(1), 1–14.

Short, J., Williams, E., & Christie, B. (1976). *The Social Psychology of Telecommunications*. Chichester: Wiley & Sons.

Sidnell, J. (2009). Comparative perspectives in Conversation Analysis. In J. Sidnell (ed.), *Conversation Analysis: Comparative perspectives* (pp. 3–27). Cambridge University Press. https://doi.org/10.1017/CBO9780511635670

Skinner, R., Napier, J., & Braun, S. (2018). Interpreting via video link: Mapping the field. In J. Napier, R. Skinner, & S. Braun (Eds), *Here or There: Research on Interpreting via Video Link* (pp. 11–39). Washington, DC: Gallaudet University Press.

Silverman, D. (1987). *Communication and Medical Practice: Social Relations in the Clinic*. London: Sage.

Spinolo, N. (2018). Traditional face-to-face telephone-mediated communication – With an interpreter. In A. Amato, N. Spinolo, & M. J. González Rodriguez (Eds), *Handbook of Remote Interpreting* (pp. 72–78). Shift in Orality Erasmus + Project: Shaping the Interpreters of the Future and of Today. <https://www.shiftinorality.eu/es/resources/2018/05/11/shift-handbook-remote-interpreting>.

Spinolo, N., Bertozzi, M., & Russo, M. (2018a). Shaping the interpreters of the future and of today: Preliminary results of the SHIFT project. *The Interpreter's Newsletter*, 23, 45–61. doi: 10.13137/2421-714X/22398

Spinolo, N., Bertozzi, M., & Russo, M. (2018b). Basic tenets and features characterizing telephone- and video-based remote communication in dialogue interpreting. In A. Amato, N. Spinolo, & M. J. González Rodriguez (Eds), *Handbook of Remote Interpreting* (pp. 12–25). Shift in Orality Erasmus + Project: Shaping the Interpreters of the Future and of Today. <https://www.shiftinorality.eu/es/resources/2018/05/11/shift-handbook-remote-interpreting>.

Stivers, T., & Robinson, J. D. (2006). A preference for progressivity in interaction. *Language in Society*, 35(3), 367–392. <https://doi.org/10.1017/S0047404506060179>.

Stivers, T., & Sidnell, J. (2005). Introduction: Multi-modal interaction. *Semiotica*, 156(1 4), 1–20. <https://doi.org/10.1515/semi.2005.2005.156.1>.

Swales, J. M. (1990). *Genre Analysis – English in Academic and Research Settings*. Cambridge: Cambridge University Press.

Tang, J., & Isaacs, E. (1993). Why do users like video?: Studies of a multimedia-supported collaboration. *Computer-supported Co-operative Work*, 1, 163–195. doi: 10.1007/BF00752437

Tannen, D. (1984). *Conversational Style*. Norwood, NJ: Ablex.

Tebble, H. (1993). A discourse model for dialogue interpreting. In *AUSIT Proceedings of the First Practitioners' Seminar* (pp. 1–26). Canberra: Australian Institute for interpreters and Translators.

Tebble, H. (1999). The tenor of consultant physicians: Implications for medical interpreting. *The Translator, 5*, 179–200. doi: 10.1080/13556509.1999.10799040

Tebble, H. (2012). Interpreting of interfering? In C. Baraldi & L. Gavioli (Eds), *Coordinating Participation in Dialogue Interpreting* (pp. 23–44). Amsterdam: John Benjamins. doi: 10.1075/btl.102.02teb

Tebble, H. (2014). A genre-based approach to teaching dialogue interpreting: The medical consultation. *The Interpreter and Translator Trainer, 8*(3), 418–436. doi: 10.1080/1750399X.2014.972651

Thiéry, C. (1976). Note on the UNESCO "Symphonie Satellite" interpretation experiment. Unpublished internal note. *Interpreting, 8*(1), 45–66. doi: 10.1075/intp.8.1.04mou

Tipton, R., & Furmanek, O. (2016). *Dialogue Interpreting: A Guide to Interpreting in Public Services and the Community*. London: Routledge. doi: 10.4324/9781315644578

Tommola, J., & Lindholm, J. (1995). Experimental research on interpreting: Which dependent variable? In J. Tommola (Ed.), *Topics in Interpreting Research* (pp. 121–133). Turku: University of Turku Press.

Valero Garcés, C. (2005). Doctor-patient consultations in dyadic and triadic exchanges. *Interpreting, 7*(2), 193–210. doi: 10.1075/intp.7.2.04val

Van der Kleij, S. (2015). *Interaction in Dutch Asylum Interviews. A Corpus Study of Interpreter-mediated Institutional Discourse*. Utrecht: Lot.

Van Dijk, T. A. (1997). *Discourse as Social Interaction*. London: Sage.

Verrept, H. (2011). Intercultural mediation through the internet in Belgian hospitals. *4th International Conference on Public Service Interpreting and Translation*, 13–15 April. <http://tisp2011.tucongreso.es/ti2011/files/book-abstracts.pdf>.

Verrept, H., & Coune, I. (2016). *Guide for Intercultural Mediation in Healthcare*. Brussels: Federale overheidsdienst Volksgezondheid, veiligheid van de voedselketen en leefmilieu – Cel interculturele bemiddeling & beleidsondersteuning. <https://www.health.belgium.be/sites/default/files/uploads/fields/fpshealth_theme_file/en_2016_04_20_leidraad.pdf>.

Verrept, H., Coune, I., Van de Velde, J., & Baatout, S. (2018). *Evaluatie projecten interculturele bemiddeling via videoconferentie*. Brussels: Research report Federale overheidsdienst Volksgezondheid, veiligheid van de voedselketen en leefmilieu – Cel interculturele bemiddeling & beleidsondersteuning. <https://www.health.belgium.be/nl/evaluatierapport-2018-interculturele-bemiddeling-op-afstand-videoconferentie>.

Vranjes, J. (2018). *On the Role of Eye Gaze in the Coordination of Interpreter-mediated Interactions an Eye-tracking Study*. PhD thesis. Leuven: University of Leuven. <https://lirias.kuleuven.be/retrieve/525192>.

Vranjes, J., Bot, H., Feyaerts, K., & Brône, G. (2019). Affiliation in interpreter-mediated therapeutic talk: On the relationship between gaze and head nods. *Interpreting*, *21*(2), 220–244. doi: 10.1075/intp.00028.vra

Wang, J. (2017). "Telephone interpreting should be used only as a last resort." Interpreters' perceptions of the suitability, remuneration and quality of telephone interpreting. *Perspectives*, *26*(1), 100–116. doi: 10.1080/0907676X.2017.1321025

Wadensjö, C. (1998). *Interpreting as Interaction*. London: Longman.

Wadensjö, C. (1999). Telephone interpreting and the synchronization of talk in social interaction. *The Translator*, *5*(2), 247–264. doi: 10.1080/13556509.1999.10799043

Wang, J., & Fang, J. (2019). Accuracy in telephone interpreting and on-site interpreting. *Interpreting*, *21*(1), 36–60. doi: 10.1075/intp.00019.wan

Warnicke, C., & Plejert, C. (2016). The positioning and bimodal mediation of the interpreter in a Video Relay Interpreting (VRI) service setting. *Interpreting*, *18*(2), 198–230. doi: 10.1075/intp.18.2.03war

Whittaker, S., & O'Connaill, B. (1997). The role of vision in face-to-face and mediated communication. In K. Finn, A. Sellen, & S. Wilbur (Eds), *Video-mediated Communication* (pp. 23–49). Mahwah, NJ: Lawrence Erlbaum.

Wofford, J. L., Campos, C. L., Johnson, D. A., & Brown, M. T. (2012). Providing a Spanish interpreter using low-cost videoconferencing in a community health centre: A pilot study using tablet computers. *Informatics in Primary Care*, *20*(2), 141–146. doi: 10.14236/jhi.v20i2.34

Xudong, D. (2009). Listener response. In S. D'hondt, J. Östman, & J. Verschueren (Eds), *The Pragmatics of Interaction* (pp. 104–124). Amsterdam: John Benjamins. doi: 10.1075/hoph.4

Young, R., & Lee, J. (2004). Identifying units in interaction: Reactive tokens in Korean and English conversations. *Journal of Sociolinguistics*, *8*(3), 380–407. doi: 10.1111/j.1467-9841.2004.00266.x

Ziegler, K., & Gigliobianco, S. (2018). Present? Remote? Remotely present! New technological approaches to remote simultaneous conference interpreting. In C. Fantinuoli (Ed.), *Interpreting and Technology* (pp. 119–139). Berlin: Language Science Press. doi: 10.5281/zenodo.1493299

Index

accuracy 9, 11, 25–26, 29, 30, 36, 38, 39, 44, 59, 61–63, 66, 106, 195, 214, 216
adjacency pairs 64, 97, 99
AIIC (Association Internationale des Interprètes de Conférence) 5, 16–18, 30, 236
alienation 19, 20, 22, 48–49
authentic data 10, 36, 48, 51, 62–63, 75, 237, 239

backchannels 34, 42, 87, 88, 92–93, 97, 141, 145, 150, 216, 218–219, 212, 222–223, 226, 227, 229
body posture 67–68, 88, 93, 161, 223
business interpreting 9, 40–41, 77, 212

chunking 51–52, 210
clients 5, 8, 21, 28, 39, 49, 54, 69, 231
code of conduct 30, 49, 90, 150, 152, 228
cognition 9, 23, 33, 42, 59, 225
  cognitive complexity 21, 43
  cognitive load 20, 54, 151, 155, 158, 176, 239
  cognitive overload *see* cognitive load
collaboration 11, 12, 17, 52, 64, 71, 133, 163, 169, 177, 182, 184, 226, 227
communication
  bilingual healthcare 12, 13, 59, 70, 71, 212, 229
  breakdown 52, 133, 134, 191, 192, 193, 218, 220, 221, 229, 231
  channels 4, 41, 191, 192, 235
  doctor–patient *see* doctor–patient consultations
  exclusion 203, 205
  flow *see* communication smoothness
  goals 42, 46, 55, 63, 66, 69, 91, 128
  issues *see* communication problems
  problems 11, 12, 70, 90, 126, 128, 234, 240
  smoothness 44–45, 51, 67, 89, 93, 94, 109, 124, 135, 144, 149–151, 159, 165, 167, 169, 172, 176–177, 182, 184–185, 188, 190, 192–193, 198–199, 220–221, 224–227, 228–229, 233–235, 239
  successfulness 55, 67, 69, 71–72, 135, 137, 157, 175, 192, 220, 224–226, 234–235, 239
  technology 3, 8, 22
community interpreting *see* dialogue interpreting
complaints
  physical 19, 21, 22, 54, 77
  psychological 19, 21, 22, 23, 54
computer-assisted interpreting 4
conference interpreting 5, 15, 18, 20–21, 23, 59, 60, 65, 205, 212
  remote 5, 15–23, 29, 30, 31, 49, 231, 236
confirmation language *see* meta communication
consecutive interpreting 3, 5, 11, 24, 27, 28, 29–31, 33, 36, 40, 48, 70, 73, 74
  remote *see* dialogue interpreting remote
conversation analysis 64, 96, 98, 162

coordination 34, 39, 60, 61, 64, 66, 67, 68, 218, 223
court interpreting *see* legal interpreting
COVID-19 pandemic 3, 7, 40
cues 62
    contextualization 33, 53, 224
    multimodal 35, 40, 62, 228
    nonverbal *see* multimodality
    paralinguistic *see* multimodality
    visual 45, 157, 189, 222, 229, 232

deaf 53–54
dialogue interpreting 5, 34, 40–42, 51, 60, 65, 150, 157, 205, 213, 222, 229, 235
    remote 5–6, 13, 15, 23, 24, 30, 54, 59
digital platforms 235
digital skills 8
digitalization 22
discourse analysis 64, 213
discourse framework 96
discourse-based approach 11, 60, 63–65, 67–68, 70, 98
doctor-patient consultations 10, 13, 63, 69, 74, 75, 95, 212
doctor-patient interaction *see* doctor-patient consultations
doctor-patient relationships *see* rapport
DUTT (Developing the Use of Technical Tools for Cross-Border Resettlement) 43–45, 47

editorialization 89, 115, 122, 158, 170–171, 205, 206, 215
efficacy 30, 36, 228, 240
efficiency 26, 41, 47, 50, 52, 54, 98, 116, 168
    cost-efficiency 42, 191, 211
ELAN 84, 98, 191
embodied communication *see* embodiment

embodied resources *see* embodiment
embodiment 51–52, 54, 98, 136–139, 145, 190, 223
empathy 62, 99, 114, 117, 120, 136–137, 156, 221–222, 229
European Union
    e-Justice 42
    European Commission 17, 43
    European Council 17
    European Court of Justice 17
    European Digital Agenda 8
    European Directive 2010/64/EU 8
    European Parliament 17, 20
experiments 8, 16–17, 20–21, 27–28, 34, 42–44, 48, 54, 76, 83, 207, 209, 211, 237, 239

fatigue 16–20, 22, 37, 44, 54, 78, 80, 155, 207
feedback *see* backchannelling

gaze 51, 67–68, 88, 93, 98, 136, 137–139, 140–141, 143–144, 153–154, 172, 173, 174, 184–186, 221–223, 231, 237
genre 69, 95
globalization 22
guidelines 13, 44–45, 50, 65

Handbook of Bilingual Videoconferencing 45
Handbook of Conference Interpreting 23
Handbook of Remote Interpreting 33, 40, 232
healthcare
    access to 24, 26, 65
    communication 12, 13, 59, 61, 69–71, 74, 96, 211–212, 233, 238
    interpreting 9, 11, 12, 13, 24, 41, 47, 60, 63, 69–70, 73, 77, 94, 158, 206, 213, 221, 239

Index   265

  policy makers 13, 235
  providers 9, 12, 24, 25, 26, 27, 28, 30,
      31, 49, 50, 54, 70–71, 96, 213, 235
human factors 19, 22, 23, 239–240

informal interpreting 25, 26, 28, 65, 77
interaction
  interactional behavior 71, 135, 138,
      149, 165, 169, 175, 177, 182, 216,
      220–224, 225, 228, 234, 235
  interactional dynamics 12, 23, 43, 51,
      54, 73, 82, 86, 91, 128, 132, 151
  interactional harmony 67
  interactional negotiation 70
  interpersonal dynamics 71, 213
interpreter ethics 62, 239
interpreter training 14, 26, 27, 34, 40,
      43–46, 50, 51, 52, 55, 77, 106, 157,
      210, 211, 215, 233–236, 239
interpreting services 4, 7–8, 11, 54,
      65, 235
interpreting style 62, 69, 81, 82, 131, 158,
      175, 177, 178–180, 202, 206, 207,
      209–210, 215, 219, 225, 233, 234
ISO standards 17, 236

language barriers 24–25
legal contexts 8, 9, 43, 46, 47
legal interpreting 9, 41, 42–47, 51,
      206, 212
liaison interpreting *see* dialogue
      interpreting

machine interpreting 4
medical communication *see* healthcare
      communication
medical interpreting *see* healthcare
      interpreting
medical studies 9, 24–32, 47, 73, 75, 77,
      87, 211, 212, 229, 230

meta communication 34, 35, 44, 128,
      150–151, 176, 218, 227
micro-analysis 9, 38, 41, 52, 102
mobile eye-tracking 67
monitoring 12, 22, 42, 67, 68, 158, 177,
      222, 225, 226, 234
monolingual communication 41,
      67, 91, 96
multimodality 12, 13, 41, 46, 51–52,
      67–68, 70, 83, 86, 98, 115, 128, 213,
      219, 227, 228, 236–237
mutual understanding 70, 71, 91, 97, 99,
      135, 142, 149, 150, 159, 163, 166,
      175, 177, 182, 198, 213, 218, 221,
      222, 226–227, 228, 229, 235,
      240

neutrality 37, 49, 191, 203, 204–205
non-professional interpreting *see* informal interpreting
non-renditions 62, 63, 66, 97

paralinguistic features 62, 88, 109
participation format 98
participation framework 64
participation status 47
patient empowerment *see* patient
      participation
patient participation 99, 101, 114, 119
patient satisfaction 9, 13, 14, 25
pragmatics 23, 32, 62, 213
process overhead *see* meta
      communication
professional code *see* code of conduct
professional interpreting 8, 25, 26, 31, 42,
      55, 71, 76, 77, 120, 172, 185, 216,
      217, 228, 239
prosody 34, 52, 68, 86, 88
public service interpreting *see* dialogue
      interpreting

qualified interpreting *see* professional interpreting
quality
    image 16, 17, 18, 50, 51, 53, 72, 88, 94, 184, 191, 197
    interpreting 8, 13, 17, 20, 28, 43, 55, 59–69, 71, 86, 111, 213, 214, 231
    of care 9, 23, 24, 26, 50, 106, 190, 191, 193, 196, 198, 199, 201, 211
    sound 27, 33, 36, 37, 39, 50, 51, 53, 72, 88, 94, 103, 104, 105, 134–135, 137, 141–142, 144–145, 146, 148, 149, 154–155, 174, 176, 180–182, 184, 185, 190, 191, 195, 197, 199, 200, 204, 218, 219, 221, 222, 224, 226, 227, 230, 234, 237

rapport 30–31, 52, 61, 96, 133, 156, 174, 176, 200, 202, 228–233
    rapport-building 44, 99, 218–219, 229–234, 238
reported speech 34, 36, 37, 38, 48, 88, 90, 92, 123, 125–126, 127, 150, 165, 167–168, 170–171, 173, 179

self-concept 228, 232, 234
Shift in Orality 32, 34, 235
simulated patient 76, 77–78, 79, 106, 213, 238
simultaneous interpreting 3, 5, 24, 27, 33, 48

remote conference interpreting, remote
social interaction 18, 60, 70
sociolinguistics 23, 60, 64
stakeholders 12, 45, 228, 235, 236
stress 16, 17, 18, 19, 20, 26, 47, 118, 135, 151, 154, 168, 175, 182, 183, 194, 200, 207, 208–209, 226, 236

technology 3–4, 5, 8, 9, 12, 13, 16, 21, 24, 27, 42, 43, 45–48, 51, 54, 74, 87, 88, 94, 101, 145, 145, 175, 190, 194, 197, 200, 214, 217, 230, 236, 239, 240
technology-mediated *see* technology
transcriptions 62, 76, 84–86, 100, 105, 115, 126
transition-relevance place 67, 148, 221
triadic communication *see* triadic exchanges
triadic constellations *see* triadic exchanges
triadic exchanges 24, 60, 65, 95, 96, 198
triangulation 11, 14, 105, 106
turn-taking 33, 34, 42, 44, 45, 5164, 65, 66, 67, 70, 82, 91, 94, 97, 128, 135, 138, 149, 162, 163, 165, 177, 220, 223, 224, 226, 233

virtual reality 21, 22
visibility 49, 52, 54, 193, 204
visual ecology 47, 228

New Trends in Translation Studies

In today's globalised society, translation and interpreting are gaining visibility and relevance as a means to foster communication and dialogue in increasingly multicultural and multilingual environments. Practised since time immemorial, both activities have become more complex and multifaceted in recent decades, intersecting with many other disciplines. *New Trends in Translation Studies* is an international series with the main objectives of promoting the scholarly study of translation and interpreting and of functioning as a forum for the translation and interpreting research community.

This series publishes research on subjects related to multimedia translation and interpreting, in their various social roles. It is primarily intended to engage with contemporary issues surrounding the new multidimensional environments in which translation is flourishing, such as audiovisual media, the internet and emerging new media and technologies. It sets out to reflect new trends in research and in the profession, to encourage flexible methodologies and to promote interdisciplinary research ranging from the theoretical to the practical and from the applied to the pedagogical.

New Trends in Translation Studies publishes translation- and interpreting-oriented books that present high-quality scholarship in an accessible, reader-friendly manner. The series embraces a wide range of publications – monographs, edited volumes, conference proceedings and translations of works in translation studies which do not exist in English. The editor, Professor Jorge Díaz Cintas, welcomes proposals from all those interested in being involved with the series. The working language of the series is English, although in exceptional circumstances works in other languages can be considered for publication. Proposals dealing with specialised translation, translation tools and technology, audiovisual translation and the field of accessibility to the media are particularly welcomed.

Vol. 1   Meng Ji: Phraseology in Corpus-Based Translation Studies
         251 pages. 2010. ISBN 978-3-03911-550-1

Vol. 2   Josu Barambones Zubiria: Mapping the Dubbing
         Scene: Audiovisual Translation in Basque Television
         191 pages. 2012. ISBN 978-3-0343-0281-4

Vol. 3   Elisa Ghia: Subtitling Matters: New Perspectives on Subtitling
         and Foreign Language Learning
         234 pages. 2012. ISBN 978-3-0343-0843-4

Vol. 4   Anabel Borja Albi and Fernando Prieto Ramos (eds): Legal
         Translation in Context: Professional Issues and Prospects
         325 pages. 2013. ISBN 978-3-0343-0284-5

Vol. 5   Kieran O'Driscoll: Retranslation through the Centuries: Jules
         Verne in English
         302 pages. 2011. ISBN 978-3-0343-0236-4

Vol. 6   Federico M. Federici (ed.): Translating Dialects and Languages
         of Minorities: Challenges and Solutions
         245 pages. 2011. ISBN 978-3-0343-0178-7

Vol. 7   Silvia Bruti and Elena Di Giovanni (eds): Audiovisual
         Translation across Europe: An Ever-changing Landscape
         289 pages. 2012. ISBN 978-3-0343-0953-0

Vol. 8   Tong-King Lee: Translating the Multilingual City: Cross-lingual
         Practices and Language Ideology
         176 pages. 2013. ISBN 978-3-0343-0850-2

Vol. 9   Laura Incalcaterra McLoughlin, Marie Biscio and Máire Áine
         Ní Mhainnín (eds): Audiovisual Translation. Subtitles and
         Subtitling: Theory and Practice
         301 pages. 2011. ISBN 978-3-0343-0299-9

Vol. 10   Xiaohui Yuan: Politeness and Audience Response in
         Chinese–English Subtitling
         250 pages. 2012. ISBN 978-3-0343-0732-1

Vol. 11 Isabel García-Izquierdo and Esther Monzó (eds): Iberian Studies on Translation and Interpreting
401 pages. 2012. ISBN 978-3-0343-0815-1

Vol. 12 Claire Ellender: Preserving Polyphonies: Translating the Writings of Claude Sarraute
250 pages. 2013. ISBN 978-3-0343-0940-0

Vol. 13 Pilar Sánchez-Gijón, Olga Torres-Hostench and Bartolomé Mesa-Lao (eds): Conducting Research in Translation Technologies
329 pages. 2015. ISBN 978-3-0343-0994-3

Vol. 14 Claire Ellender: Dealing with Difference in Audiovisual Translation: Subtitling Linguistic Variation in Films
221 pages. 2015. ISBN 978-3-0343-1816-7

Vol. 15 Anna Jankowska and Agnieszka Szarkowska (eds): New Points of View on Audiovisual Translation and Media Accessibility
316 pages. 2015. ISBN 978-3-0343-1842-6

Vol. 16 Charlotte Bosseaux: Dubbing, Film and Performance: Uncanny Encounters
251 pages. 2015. ISBN 978-3-0343-0235-7

Vol. 17 Guadalupe Soriano-Barabino: Comparative Law for Legal Translators
220 pages. 2016. ISBN 978-3-0343-1725-2

Vol. 18 Şebnem Susam-Saraeva: Translation and Popular Music: Transcultural Intimacy in Turkish–Greek Relations
184 pages. 2015. ISBN 978-3-03911-887-8

Vol. 19 Celia Martín de León and Víctor González-Ruiz (eds): From the Lab to the Classroom and Back Again: Perspectives on Translation and Interpreting Training
371 pages. 2016. ISBN 978-3-0343-1985-0

Vol. 20   Carla Mereu Keating: The Politics of Dubbing: Film Censorship and State Intervention in the Translation of Foreign Cinema in Fascist Italy
191 pages. 2016. ISBN 978-3-0343-1838-9

Vol. 21   Susanne M. Cadera and Andrew Samuel Walsh (eds): Literary Retranslation in Context
252 pages. 2017. ISBN 978-3-0343-1996-6

Vol. 22   Kayoko Nohara: Translating Popular Fiction: Embracing Otherness in Japanese Translations
248 pages. 2018. ISBN 978-3-0343-1963-8

Vol. 23   Pierre-Alexis Mével: Subtitling African American English into French: Can We *Do the Right Thing*?
256 pages. 2017. ISBN 978-3-0343-1897-6

Vol. 24   Micòl Beseghi: Multilingual Films in Translation: A Sociolinguistic and Intercultural Study of Diasporic Films
256 pages. 2017. ISBN 978-1-78707-159-9

Vol. 25   Michal Borodo: Translation, Globalization and Younger Audiences: The Situation in Poland
248 pages. 2017. ISBN 978-1-78707-473-6

Vol. 26   Eugenia Dal Fovo and Paola Gentile (eds): Translation and Interpreting: Convergence, Contact and Interaction
308 pages. 2019. ISBN 978-1-78707-750-8

Vol. 27   Nana Sato-Rossberg and Akiko Uchiyama (eds): Diverse Voices in Translation Studies in East Asia
224 pages. 2019. ISBN 978-178874-022-7

Vol. 28   Sarah M. A. Reed: Translating Cultural Identity: French Translations of Australian Crime Fiction
260 pages. 2019. ISBN 978-1-78874-007-4

Vol. 29   Blanca Arias-Badia: Subtitling Television Series: A Corpus-Driven Study of Police Procedurals
274 pages. 2020. ISBN 978-1-78707-796-6

Vol. 30 Károly Polcz: Speech Acts, Directness and Politeness in
        Dubbing: American Television Series in Hungary
        270 pages. 2020. ISBN 978-1-78874-232-0

Vol. 31 María Dolores Rodríguez Melchor, Ildikó Horváth
        and Kate Ferguson (eds): The Role of Technology in
        Conference Interpreter Training
        262 pages. 2020. ISBN 978-1-78874-407-2

Vol. 32 Ali Almanna and Juan Jose Martinez Sierra (eds):
        Reframing Realities through Translation
        300 pages. 2020. ISBN 978-1-78997-228-3

Vol. 33 Alícia Moreno Giménez: The Translation of Irony: Examining
        its Translatability into Narratives
        262 pages. 2022. ISBN 978-1-78997-984-8

Vol. 34 Esther de Boe: Remote Interpreting in Healthcare Settings
        290 pages. 2023. ISBN 978-1-80079-373-6

www.ingramcontent.com/pod-product-compliance
Ingram Content Group UK Ltd.
Pitfield, Milton Keynes, MK11 3LW, UK
UKHW021829140426
5217IPUK00017B/1266